Advance Praises for
Portraits of Huntington's

"When thinking about Huntington's Disease, it is difficult to avoid dwelling on the many negative consequences this terrible disease has for the individual and the family. *Portraits of Huntington's* helps us to find the positive side. Carmen Leal's stories are full of courage, strength, faith, love, and humor that HD families demonstrate in their everyday lives. *Portraits* is a personal book, with funny stories, touching reminiscences, and hard realities, and, like her first book, *Faces of Huntington's, Portraits* is filled with Carmen's indomitable spirit and joy. It will be a pleasure to have this book on our clinic bookshelf to offer our patients and their families."

Pat Allinson, M.S. Genetic Counselor
HD Program Coordinator University of Virginia
Medical Center

"These are tremendously important stories that needed to be told, and Carmen does so with warmth, humanity, and grace. I truly couldn't put it down until the end. Congratulations on a beautiful book."

Gary Barg. Editor-in-Chief
Today's Caregiver Magazine caregiver.com

"This is a heart-warming, powerful book that will have a tremendous impact on those whose lives have been affected by Huntington's Disease, and an inspiration to anyone who values human courage and strength."

Barbara T. Boyle, National Executive Director/CEO,
Huntington's Disease Society of America, Inc.

"*Portraits of Huntington's* is a wonderful collection of stories about people who are affected in some way by Huntington's Disease. Although it can be read a little bit at a time, I found I could not put it down. I laughed. I cried. I was inspired. I highly recommend it for anyone with an interest in Huntington's Disease, as well as for those who are not familiar with HD."

Renette Davis - Librarian,
Huntington's Disease Information Webmaster

"Having been at risk for Huntington's Disease for many decades, and having been active for exactly 25 years in the Dutch Huntington Society and the International Huntington Association supporting HD families, I experienced and learned that recognition is an extremely important part of coping with the threat of and live with Huntington's Disease. Portraits of Huntington's will help those affected in one way or another by HD to learn that they are not the only one's in the world with their distress, fear and loneliness. With understanding, love, humour and a will to fight, a life with HD is a life worth living."

Gerrit R. Dommerholt
International Development Officer and
former President of the International Huntington Association

"*Portraits of Huntington's* is a book of lessons in living life to the fullest. You will learn first hand about true courage in the face of the challenges of HD. The book is finished; yet the memories remain, and these brave souls now have a place in my heart. Their stories lead me to reaffirm my intention to live a joyful life!"

Carol Levenson, RN, MS
HD Nurse Consultant, Family Caregiver Alliance

"I experienced the gamut of emotions while reading *Portraits of Huntington's*. I laughed at some bits, cried at some (well there were tears in my eyes), and was made to think of others. This book accomplishes what it sets out to be—basically, Portraits of Huntington's."

Ron Livingstone
Chairman, Scottish Huntington's Association

"I loved reading *Portraits of Huntington's*. I only found one problem; It is too short! *Portraits of Huntington's* tells us true stories of real people, and I think that all of us can find our feelings reflected in the book. More importantly, we can find a useful way to cope with our feelings in an upbeat and optimistic way.

"I think it is also very useful for professionals and others who have to answer so many questions each day. Huntington's families think I have got the answers, but a lot of them are in Carmen Leal's book.

"I used to say to them, without success, I might add; 'There is always something good in any situation you are facing, you only have to have the ability to find it.' Now I can suggest a book that says the same thing. *Portraits of Huntington's* teaches readers the ability to find the 'good view.'"

Asunción Martínez, President
Asociación de Corea de Huntington Española (ACHE)

"*Portraits of Huntington's* is a loving portrayal of some of the special people to be found in the Huntington's community. With her stories of people with the disease and those who care for them, Carmen Leal shows that while Huntington's changes lives and results in grievous losses, the world is a better place for the strength, determination, humor, and love shown by each of these special people. I have been fortunate enough to meet several of the people whose stories are told so beautifully in this book; others I can never know, but thanks to Carmen, I will forget none of them and continue to learn from their examples."

Marsha L. Miller, Ph.D.
Huntington's Disease Advocacy Center
http://www.hdac.org

"I had to speak to two hundred nurses at a recent study day. I asked a person with Huntington's to tell me what she would like me to tell the group on her behalf. Her physical symptoms are severe, but she is very alert. It took a while for her to give a clear answer, but it was worth the wait.

'Tell them to stop treating me as if I'm a fool, and tell them to keep out of my way when I'm trying to do the bit I am able to do.' Their memory is intact, their eyes express their ability, but, are we listening?

"I love Carmen's book because it forces us to look at the person behind the label of HD, and it reminds us that the person with Huntington's is not always the one with the emotional problems! This book is a great way to give people with Huntington's a voice."

Bernadette Moran, Development Officer
Huntington's Disease Association of Ireland

"*Portraits of Huntington's* offers many fresh new insights into the devastating realities of Huntington's Disease. But, more importantly, Carmen Leal's new book conveys an inspirational message of joy. It reveals the special role that humour, perseverance, and faith can play in surviving— even thriving—in the face of adversity. By introducing us to her own family and to others who know what Huntington's Disease looks like right up close, Leal helps to break down myths and misconceptions and to build empathy and understanding. Above all, she reminds us that people with Huntington's Disease are, first and foremost, people."

Rod Morrison, D. Phil., Executive Director,
Huntington Society of Canada

"Carmen has masterfully interwoven personal anecdotal stories with touching HD testimonials. This book is a riveting tapestry evidencing lives which triumph over the tragedy that HD produces.

"This book deserves a wide audience, both inside and outside the HD community. In *Portraits of Huntington's,* Carmen has taken the lemon of HD and made lemonade. She reminds us of the indomitable human spirit.

I am proud to have Carmen as a friend, who gently grafted me into the HD family. For that, I will be eternally grateful."

Marie Nemec, Three time bicyclist across America
for HD fundraising and awareness

To Rosilyn,
wishing
you joy &
happiness.
Aloha,
Carmen

$\mathscr{P}$ortraits
of $\mathscr{H}$untington's

CHOOSING JOY THROUGH
LIFE LESSONS

CARMEN LEAL
With Portraits by Ruth Hargrave

Essence
PUBLISHING

Belleville, Ontario, Canada

Portraits of Huntington's

Copyright © 2001, Carmen Leal

"This Joy I Have" is written by Merrill Leal. Used by permission.

"Pinches of Salt, Prisms of Light" and "Endless Dreams" are written by Soon Hee Newbold Rettig. Used by permission of Blue Fire Productions.

ISBN: 1-55306-251-5

Essence Publishing is a Christian Book Publisher dedicated to furthering the work of Christ through the written word. For more information, contact: 44 Moira Street West, Belleville, Ontario, Canada K8P 1S3.
Phone: 1-800-238-6376. Fax: (613) 962-3055.
E-mail: info@essencegroup.com
Internet: www.essencegroup.com

Printed in Canada
by

Essence
PUBLISHING

To David Pock, who many of you met in Faces of Huntington's.
I hope you enjoy getting to know him even better in this book.
Thank you, Dave, for being my Sacrifice Fly.

Table of Contents

Knowledge

Laughter

Patience

Compassion

Faith

Love

Hope

Joy

Acknowledgements

In my life, choosing joy only became possible when I understood that God first chose me. Knowing that I am loved by God, knowing that He sacrificed His Son for me, makes my life not just easier to live, but joyful, too. So first I acknowledge and thank God for His overwhelming love.

What would I do without Ruth Hargrave? Not only is she the wonderful artist who contributed so much to this book, she is also my friend. I value her strength, humor, compassion, and deep faith.

Choosing Jim Pollard to write the foreword and featuring him in this book was an easy decision. Jim, you are hereby served notice: You will never be allowed to leave the Huntington's movement until there is a cure and until everyone who needs care has received it. You are *truly* a special person—and a much loved one, I might add.

When I signed on to the Internet so many years ago, I never dreamed of the difference it would make in my life and the lives of so many others. Thank you to the countless Huntington's friends over the years from HDCaregivers, Hunt-Dis, and various chat rooms and forums.

How can I ever thank my dear friend and editor, JoAnn Zarling? JoAnn believed in me long before I really believed I could write a book. She graciously and gently polished my words, not only for this book, but for *Faces of Huntington's* as well. JoAnn, your friendship and support, despite your own physical challenges, inspire and humble me.

Foreword

When life delivers those proverbial lemons, some people choose to make lemonade. Some joyful spirits with an ample supply of lemons make several pitchers of lemonade—enough for everyone. And a few brave souls make a lemon spice cake using the whole lemon, including the grated rinds!

Portraits of Huntington's is a book about these joyous folk. For them, Huntington's Disease provides an apparently unlimited supply of lemons. You may have another lemon provider—Parkinson's, Hodgkin's, Alzheimer's, or one of the myriad handicapping diseases of the body. Perhaps your lemons come by way of financial, marital, or career problems. No matter from where you're supplied, this is a book about choosing joy, regardless of what you face, regardless of what is on your horizon.

This is a book about life, about living life with a lemon and squeezing it until you've extracted every last drop of available joy. It's about wringing it tighter still because you're confident that there's still another drop in there somewhere.

For the last two decades, I've been uniquely positioned to spend time with people, with whole families, who are presented with supreme challenges. Some challenges affect only one, while others touch the lives of everyone in the family and even those around it. Some challenges last for decades, lifetimes, or even generations. Mostly, they have involved the extended care of family members in their own households and in nursing homes. All of these challenges have profoundly affected their lives and have even defined who they are.

I have had to watch as some families choose to ignore their challenges only to be torn apart by them sooner or later. Some families simply endure the losses that come part-and-parcel with everything, struggling one day at a time until the days become weeks, months, and finally long years. Those who endure, though, are those who choose to sift through the rubble with which these challenges litter their lives until they find the gifts. Yes, there are gifts. Unfortunately, relatively few choose to look for them among the shattered fragments left by some of life's toughest battles.

Portraits of Huntington's is a book about those who never seem to stop looking for gifts. After all, sometimes it takes unimaginable strength to keep looking. On the surface, it's a book about the wonderful people who deliberately opt to look on the "bright side" as their families face debilitating illness. Essentially, though, it's about how great human spirits can conquer whatever life places in their way... if they so choose.

As chance would have it, the conquering spirits I am most familiar with all have Huntington's Disease. I have watched as, after decades of struggle, they still make the daily choice to find the joy around them. Surely, it's not easy. For years, they feared the onset of subtle symptoms. They looked forward and saw loss after loss: their jobs, their driving, friends, family members, etc. I know they struggle to go on and often find themselves in the thick of the battle—but it's a battle they *choose* to fight. Or so I thought. Now, after years of watching many fight a multitude of battles, it has become apparent that it's not a "battle" they're fighting, after all.

HD, PD, AD, bad luck, no luck, unfathomable losses... now I see that life's lemons are not enemy attacks. It's not a battle at all! The nuance of "battle" is significantly different than "struggle." You *battle* a foe in wartime; you *struggle* with circumstances in order to overcome. Though subtle, the difference in meaning is monumental to me.

Even for those who have actively chosen joy, it can be a progressively difficult struggle to find the wonder and pleasure in the next hour or the next day. Often, it grows more difficult each moment to find the positive in the now or commonplace, in what's at hand or what lies ahead. The life that was so frightening from afar is now a day-to-day choice, and still, each and every day, these strugglers choose to look for joy. As difficult as it gets, they try again because they learn something new every day. Their pervading motto is "try even harder tomorrow," colored by the humor of the realization that it can't really get any worse!

But this is where that so-subtle difference between words expands to gargantuan proportions; another loss is not a surrender as it would be in a battle. Loss is just a matter of pulling up stakes to prospect for the gifts in a more promising spot. The strugglers' gain in claiming this positive attitude is revealed to them today, and it is enough to launch another search tomorrow.

17

Are you in need of a second wind in your own struggles? Then look at these portraits of Huntington's. You've heard about "the indomitable human spirit." It will be found within the pages of this wonderful book.

Jim Pollard
2001

Preface

Probably the most frequently asked question since the release of my first book, *Faces of Huntington's,* has been, "When are you going to write another book?"

At first, I just shuddered and said, "Never! It's too much work!"

But so many readers wrote and emailed about how *Faces of Huntington's* had impacted either their own lives or the lives of those they knew, that gradually, I began warming to the idea. This time, though, I wanted to produce a book that did more than reach out to the HD community. I wanted it to educate "outsiders" about Huntington's.

"Who did the cover?" That's the second most common question about *Faces of Huntington's.* By now, if you've read the book, you know that I designed it to coordinate with stories about both the shoes and the kites that appear on the cover. The boats were the brainchild of Ruth Hargrave, who painted the picture and added them as a tribute to her son who has HD.

Ruth is a gifted artist and a full-time caregiver. Sadly, after the death of her husband, three of her four children have tested positive for the Huntington's gene, and two of them are symptomatic. Despite the grief she lives with each day, she finds joy in her art. When I asked her to consider painting the cover, she said, "Well, I've never done one. I can do it though." And did she ever!

For the past six years, I have been a speaker at the Huntington's Disease Society of America's annual convention. I have also had the privilege of traveling throughout the United States to speak at Huntington's Disease conferences, at churches, and at United Way events. During these presentations, I've been able to tell many stories that aren't in *Faces of Huntington's*. There, too, people have asked me to include them in another book. But it took me a while to tackle another huge project.

Some of you may think this book is *Faces of Huntington's, Part Two*. While I'd like to one day write another book similar to *Faces of Huntington's*, this isn't it.

Ruth's incredible portraits go with many of the stories I tell. Those stories, along with some new ones, seemed to be exactly what my readers were requesting. Using joy as the book's underlying theme means there is something for everyone. Whether you or a family member has been diagnosed with HD, whether you're a caregiver, someone at risk, a professional who works with HD, or maybe just someone who cares—we all need joy in our lives. We need a counterbalance for things that go wrong. And Huntington's or not, things do go wrong.

There are tens of thousands of special people who deserve to have their portraits in books, and all of their stories need to be told. Obviously, there simply isn't room in this book. *Portraits of Huntington's* features the portraits and stories of seven special people or family groups who have Huntington's Disease. I have also included the portrait and story of one professional because our professionals are another "portrait" of this disease.

These stories, some about HD, some not, are about things that happened in my life that taught me valuable lessons. I believe we need to choose joy daily if we want it to overrule the negatives in life. When we actively pursue knowledge, laughter, patience, compassion, faith, love, and hope, we are in a better position to choose joy.

There are several stories that might seem familiar to some. These stories appeared, in slightly different form, in my book, *Pinches of Salt, Prisms of Light*. Sadly, this book is out of print at the present time. Because several stories fit into *Portraits* so well, and because few in the Huntington's community have read the book, I've included them for your enjoyment. The following stories are reprinted from *Pinches of Salt, Prisms of Light*: "A Heart As Big As Alaska," "Dave's Goofy Day," "Expressions of Love," "I'll Love You Forever," "My Job Is To Say, 'I Love You,'" "Sweetness," and "The Treasure Box."

People with Huntington's and their families are among the most courageous people I've ever known. Each year at the close of the Saturday Awards Banquet at the Huntington's Disease Society of America convention, they play the song, "We Are Family." Most of us would probably never have chosen to be a part of this particular family, but you *can* choose joy in the midst of all the challenges Huntington's gives you each day.

My hope is that these stories and portraits will be of help as you continue to look for joy in life. I also hope you will share these stories, these portraits of Huntington's, with others.

Introduction

In the foreword to *Faces of Huntington's*, Dr. Richard Dubinsky said,

> Despite all the research that has been completed and the studies still underway, Carmen's book reminds us that Huntington's Disease is not an entity in itself. It is a disease that affects people and their families and caregivers. Too often, in the practice of medicine, we lose sight of the patient because of the disease. Clinicians and researchers, as well as caregivers and family members, need to be reminded that Huntington's Disease is an illness that affects people.

Dr. Dubinsky reminds us that the disease affects the entire family, not only the people who have the gene and are symptomatic. When dealing with Huntington's, or any other chronic or terminal disease, it's all too easy to become angry, depressed, and bitter. After David was diagnosed, I decided that it would not ruin my life. I would choose joy.

Joy is a choice. Happiness is based on a set of circumstances. More often than not, since Huntington's Disease entered my life, I have not been particularly happy.

But I *have* been joyful, and joy is the motor that pushes me through.

In January 1998, two years after my family moved to Florida, my thirty-six-year-old brother died of *primary sclerosing cholangitis*. It was, and still is, difficult to imagine him not being here. He touched so many lives during his too-short time on this earth.

Merrill was a pastor with incredible wisdom for one so young. He also wrote music and had a voice that can only be described as liquid joy. Years ago, I recorded one of his songs on my first album. He wrote "This Joy I Have" at the age of seventeen while in the hospital, battling the insidious disease that eventually took his life.

The depth and truth of his words recently struck me anew. Though he didn't battle Huntington's Disease, another disease threatened to rob his joy. I can truthfully say that Merrill—and his family—kept their joy until the end, as have countless Huntington's families.

The lyrics of Merrill's song speak of a joy that comforts and brightens our days. Joy is something we must choose on a daily, if not hourly, basis. We need to have patience, knowledge, and endurance to fully experience joy—no matter the situation.

Adela Rogers St. Johns said,

> Joy seems to me a step beyond happiness—happiness is the sort of atmosphere you can live in sometimes, when you're lucky. Joy is a light that fills you with hope and faith and love.

One morning last November, while singing "This Joy I Have," I decided that the theme of *Portraits of Huntington's* would be joy. In these pages you will see portraits of incredible men and women who have also chosen joy. I hope their inspiring lives, coupled with my stories, will encourage you to choose joy, too.

"This Joy I Have"
by Merrill Leal

This joy I have is like a sweet river.
It flows down deep in my soul.
It comforts me when I am sad.
It brightens my day with peace.

This joy I have, it comes with patience
that only the Spirit can bring.
This joy I have it comes with knowledge
that can only supply what I need.

This joy I have is like a sweet river.
It flows down deep in my soul.
It takes the sorrows I used to have
and changes them into peace and love.

This joy that I have, it comes with endurance
that you only get when you serve the Lord.
This joy that I have, it comes with patience
that you only get when you obey the Lord.

This joy I have is like a sweet river.
It flows so sweet in my soul.
It comforts me when I am sad
and gives me the rest that I need.

Knowledge

---

*The essence of knowledge is:
having it, to apply it; not having it,
to confess your ignorance.*

—CONFUCIUS

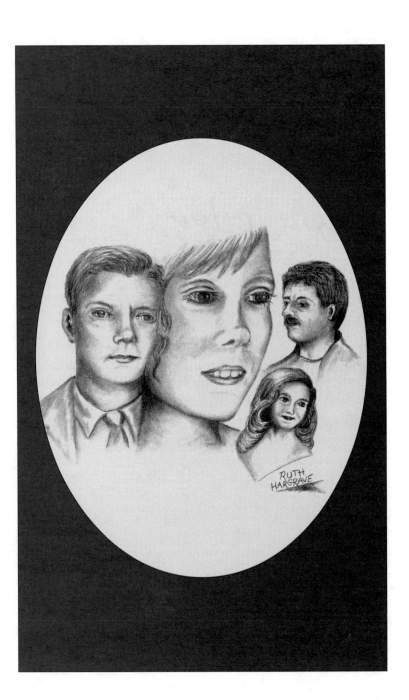

A Sense of Family

He that raises a large family does, indeed, while he lives to observe them, stand a broader mark for sorrow; but then he stands a broader mark for pleasure too.

—Benjamin Franklin

"Life is like a picture, so paint it well!" I smile when I see this signature on each of Ruth Hargrave's email messages. Ruth has made that signature her personal credo, and she follows it every day.

When asked how she can take care of so many people, Ruth explains: "I have a strong sense of family. I learned it from my mother because our lives are similar. She took care of my father, crippled in a car accident, until his death. Keeping the family together—all four children: two sons and two daughters—gave her a reason to get up each day."

Ruth and Bill were childhood sweethearts, dating throughout his four years of naval service, her high school years. Then, in 1952, Ruth became Mrs. William Hargrave III. Little did they know, by the time Bill's father died in an automobile accident, he had already bequeathed a cruel legacy—the HD gene—to his son, grandchildren, and future generations.

Within five years, Ruth and Bill were parents to four children: two boys and two girls. Their "spare" time went into building a trailer court park in upstate New York. It was hard work, but together they did all the physical labor, built up their business, raised their children, and watched their dreams grow into reality.

Twelve years later, they sold the business and moved to Virginia Beach, Virginia. There, Bill went to work for Norfolk Southern Railroad. They lived in a double-wide mobile home which allowed the family to purchase a nice motorhome. The one thing Bill truly enjoyed was traveling America in their home.

Then, in 1984, he fell from the top of a moving railroad car and lost both legs.

Bill had always been a heavy drinker. Suddenly he was forced to quit "cold turkey," which made his long hospital stay even longer. He was in the trauma unit for three months and on the regular floor for another month. After he went home, strange things began happening: his hands would fly all over, uncontrollable, with a will of their own; he had trouble sitting on the commode; even at night his strange, erratic yells made rest impossible. After thirty-five years of marriage, it seemed Ruth couldn't please her husband in any way.

At first, she thought it was the loss of his legs. Maybe, too, it was the withdrawal from all the strong medication he had been receiving. Finally, though, he grew so violent, so irrational, and his behavior so increasingly weird, that she had to have him committed. This man, whom she had loved most of her life, appeared to be gone—a monster had taken his place.

When the doctor at the hospital saw Bill bite the nurse, it triggered a thought. Perhaps, he suggested, Bill had Huntington's Disease. Eventually, Cindy, their third child, began having similar symptoms, and it seemed she, too, had HD. By the time the DNA test was available, Bill Jr., their second child, had also become symptomatic. Sadly, both children received positive results. Bill's blood was also tested, and of course, at long last, the diagnosis became a reality. All three of them had HD.

Ruth then went to the library for information but found very little available. Until her husband died in 1995, she just stumbled through caring for him in the best way she could. He didn't talk much following his diagnosis, and Ruth often wondered just what was really going on behind those large brown eyes of his.

After Bill died, Ruth focused on her daughter. Cindy had two children by this time: Christine, the eldest, and Daniel. Christine was on her own, and Daniel still needed care. Her son-in-law was long gone, so Ruth made a hard decision; she decided to take part of her savings and build an addition to her home. That way there would be a place for her HD-positive son, daughter, and at-risk grandson. It was a huge expense, but she felt it was necessary. These two adult children had no one else. The Lord had entrusted them to her.

Cindy has since progressed to the point of requiring a significant amount of attention—more than Ruth could give. "I couldn't care for her as well the rest of the family," explains Ruth. "Last year Cindy went into an assisted living facility. This past month she was having so many rages they moved her to a nursing home."

We hear every day about the poor quality of care in our nation's nursing homes, and, in some cases, it's true. For Cindy, thank goodness, the reality is quite different. "We had a meeting with the nursing home staff because she was acting up. Right now, Cindy is settling in and things are okay," says a very relieved Ruth. "I am truly impressed with this nursing home. They have bent over backwards to make it work for Cindy."

You've heard the trite phrase, "Like father like son." In the Hargrave family, this is true. Besides having HD, Ruth's son, Bill, is an alcoholic just like his father.

"It's true," agrees Ruth. "He has an alcohol problem. When Bill drinks he loses control. His last outburst got him removed from my home, and he went to the North Carolina state hospital for over a week while they reviewed his medications. Since coming home, he seems better. He knows if he has even one drink I will send him away."

While some might think this is somewhat cruel, Ruth calls it "tough love," and she's right. When Bill is drinking, Ruth cannot take care of the others under her roof, and they are family, too.

Bill finds enjoyment in his favorite past time—the CB radio. He talks to others on their way to work, naps, and talks to them on their way home. Maybe, in some way, the conversations make him feel a part of a world that he has already lost.

Ruth's third child with Huntington's, Sue, lives nearby in her own home. Her husband left her in August with the princely sum of $2 in her pocket. "Because Sue home-schooled her daughter, Jessica, for thirteen years and did not work outside the home, she doesn't qualify for disability. She is waiting to hear if she will receive any income from Social Security."

Sadly, Huntington's doesn't stop with the first generation, or one's children. In the Hargrave family, some grandchildren are already affected. Sue's oldest daughter, Tina, tested positive after experiencing symptoms while in the military in Saudi during the Gulf War. Sue's fourteen-year-old daughter, Jessica, is now with her father and, like her three siblings—C.J, Britny, and Mike—is at risk for Huntington's Disease.

So far, Ruth's fourth son, Steven, has chosen to remain untested and has no symptoms. This is great news for his two children, James and Lauren.

"This certainly isn't the life I envisioned when I was a newlywed in New York," reflects Ruth. "It's not all struggles though. Daniel, my grandson, has lived with me since 1995. I raised him through the teen years with nary a problem. He talked me into buying my first computer and taught me to use it."

Ruth is justifiably proud as she talks about Daniel's future. He's been through computer college and has two different certifications. "He is working with a young computer company and still lives with the 'Gramma' who loves him."

One would think that having three of four children and one grandchild with Huntington's would be more than any person could handle. But those who think that way haven't met Ruth Hargrave.

Ruth gets profound satisfaction when she can help one of her family members. "It's a deep feeling to be needed, and I am needed."

"I am sixty-seven years young," continues Ruth. "God blessed me with good health. He must have known the job I was facing."

If that's the case, and I believe it is, He also endowed Ruth with patience, humor, intelligence, and other qualities needed to face each day. God's provision is so complete that, in addition to Ruth's caregiving qualities, He gifted her with a wonderful talent.

Ruth is an artist. It is her portraits that grace the pages of this book. She also was the artist who took my vision and did an incredible job painting the cover of *Faces of Huntington's*.

"I have a love of art," says Ruth. "It brings me joy and helps fill spaces inside me that need filling. It also fills my home, which is beginning to look like a museum. Book cases, tables, shelves, paintings, portraits, light switches, and stones are all canvases for my art. Even the toilet seat! In the future I want to paint a mouse hole in the floor molding with a mouse looking out. I also enjoy filet crochet, which is art work with a hook. You crochet a picture which is neat."

Ruth is quick to add that she has a life apart from family. Besides belonging to the National Decorative Painters Association, she belongs to the Tidewater Decorative Painters and sits on the Currituck Senior Center board. She has earned five gold medals and one silver in seven county art competitions. Ruth is active in the Huntington Disease movement, too. She attends the local support group meetings and was a featured speaker at the national HDSA convention in Orlando and the HD Symposium in Newport News, Virginia.

"I work the polls in Currituck County; I travel, have been on numerous cruises, and visited many countries. I drive to my home in upstate New York about once a year and have been up and down the east coast. I used to love to ice skate and was in a local ice show in 1952. Age has made me hang up my skates, and now I just enjoy watching the young at it."

Ruth emphatically points to her solid Christian faith as the driving force in her life. More than anything, this carries her through the most difficult of times.

"I think God has a caregiver plan for me, and I seem to fit that place well. Sometimes I dream of sitting on the beach in Miami, in my bikini, but then I come down to earth and realize that I am truly where God wants me, and I shall try to be content and do my very best. I have learned to step back and let God do His work. I can't do it all. He can."

Amadou

If you haven't got any charity in your heart, you have the worst kind of heart trouble.

—BOB HOPE

"Madame. S'il vous plaît me donner l'argent. Il est pour mes enfants. Ils ont faim."

The claw-like hand clutched the hem of my skirt as I navigated my way back to my house. My high school French and the woman's emaciated frame were enough to help me understand her plight. Her two children, with eyes dwarfing their faces, intensified my feelings of helplessness as I trudged through the dusty streets.

Tossing a few of my dwindling francs into her bowl, I continued home. Her thanks followed me as I saw more of the same. The blind woman with no arms, the man with leprosy, and the tiny children struggling with crudely-made crutches, were only a few in the never-ending parade from hell-on-earth.

One day, before the end my second month in Mali, I went to see the Peace Corps director. "I have a problem," I explained. "In the market today, bargaining for food, I ran out of money. You guys aren't paying me enough. No matter how I try, I can't make it."

"Have you been giving money to the beggars?"

"Of course I have! How can I not? There are so many,

and each seems to have more problems than the one before."

The director then told me how every new volunteer has the same predicament. With so many needs everywhere one looked, how could we help them all? My job was to teach English at the local high school. In my zealousness to help those in need, I had given away far too great a percentage of money to the beggars, leaving nothing for myself.

"There is no way you can help every beggar in your neighborhood, let alone in the city. Why not choose one beggar to adopt? Instead of feeling guilty about what you can't do, why not think of what you *can* do that will make a difference?"

Most beggars live in a world of contempt. He suggested I choose one beggar to help and give the others a kind word or a smile. Most of these mendicants rarely had any kindness shown to them so, though it wouldn't fill their stomachs, a kindly smile, a gracious word, would still be a gift.

I chose Amadou as "my" beggar. Leprosy had eaten away half of Amadou's face. Born with no legs, one complete, though withered arm, and a stump at the elbow of the other arm, my poor friend also had *elephantiasis* of the testicles. Amadou spent his days on a large, homemade, skateboard-like contraption—a board on wheels that he operated by pushing himself along with his "good" arm.

I took the director's suggestion. At first I felt awful not giving to everyone, but eventually, I learned how best to be of benefit in Mali. My job was to teach, not to feed the hundreds of hungry people I came face-to-face with each day, no matter how much I wanted to.

Now, twenty-five years later, my first job is to be the best wife, mother, and friend I can be. When Dave became symptomatic and eventually diagnosed, I had to decide my priorities. Everything that wasn't essential was relegated to a lower level, or even eliminated. My family was where I spent my energies.

One of my priorities has been to give myself time and permission to grieve. Just as I grieved over the plight of my African friends, I lamented the changes in Dave. This was not just *his* disease, but our family's.

Taking care of myself was equally important. I realized if I didn't, I wouldn't be able to take care of anyone else.

Alice Walker says,

> Wherever I have knocked, a door opened. Wherever I have wandered, a path has appeared. I have been helped, supported, encouraged, and nurtured by people of all races, creeds, colors, and dreams.

Like Walker, I have always tried to give to others because I, too, have been given much and helped by so many.

I went to Mali to help others and, at one level, I did just that. I also learned a number of valuable lessons from the people, their situations, and my surroundings. Whenever I find myself overwhelmed with life and Huntington's, I remember Amadou. I can't write a check to fund the cure. I can't even reach out and physically touch the tens-of-thousands who need a hug. I can, however, pray for us all and touch people with my words and my music.

But I'm Scared!

Nothing in life is to be feared. It is only to be understood.

—MARIE CURIE

"But I'm scared, Mamma," cried Natalie. "I can't go to bed. If I go to sleep I'll have nightmares."

My sister, Diane, sighed as she contemplated yet another hysterical, tear-filled evening. Why did bedtime have to be so difficult every night? If it wasn't Natalie's bedtime fears, it was something else with Christina, her eldest daughter, or Chelsea, her youngest.

"I have them all the time," wailed Natalie. "I'm scared. Can't I stay down here with you and Daddy? I'll be good."

Diane knew that acquiescence was not the answer. Natalie needed to overcome her fears, not yield to them. Diane pondered the vast differences in her daughters once again. Christina was mature beyond her years, while Chelsea delighted in life as one big game. Natalie was the worrier.

"We've had this discussion before, Natalie. Staying up is not an option. You're going to sleep. Let's go. Now," added Diane, anticipating Natalie's oft-suggested plan that she sleep with her parents. "In your room. In your bed. *Now*."

Her husband, Cedric, added still more clothes to the piles of clean, folded laundry, while he calmly watched another episode in the Stein family circus. Diane threw an angry glance over her shoulder as she unsuccessfully tried to herd her three darlings upstairs. *Why didn't he do something?*

As if on cue, Cedric said, "Here, Natalie," and tossed a piece of clothing to her. Natalie nimbly caught a pair of her daddy's underwear in an outstretched hand. "Put these on. If you wear these on your head while you sleep, they'll keep out the nightmares."

Diane stared at the father of her children as if he'd lost his mind. Weren't things bad enough already?

"Is that true, Daddy?" asked six-year-old Natalie, before Diane had a chance to explain their father was just teasing.

"It certainly is, sweetheart. I promise."

For generations, little girls have trusted their daddies, and Natalie was no different.

"Okay. I'll try it." With a shrug of her shoulders and a wide grin, Natalie pulled her father's white briefs on her head, waistband first.

"I want some, too," screamed Chelsea. "I don't want nightmares either.

"Me, too," yelled Christina.

The tone of the house changed instantly, as three little girls danced around the house in their daddy's "tighty whities." All thoughts of nightmares evaporated as their shrill giggles made their way upstairs.

"I don't believe it," said my bemused sister with one last look at her husband and a shake of her head. "Whatever it takes."

"But I'm scared!" That's what Natalie genuinely felt each night at bedtime. Nightmares, even the thought of nightmares, can be very scary. Her father didn't try to convince her that she wouldn't have bad dreams. Instead, he acknowledged her fears and gave her something tangible to help her.

"But I'm scared!" That's what each of us must surely have felt when we learned about the possibility of Huntington's Disease. Who wouldn't be scared?

We've come a long way from the days when people with Huntington's symptoms were locked in mental hospitals, or worse. But the many treatments that are available today are only effective for those who are not in denial.

Unfortunately, denial is alive and well in the HD community. Denial is often a defense mechanism, and it can be healthy—to a point. Beyond that point, however, it is most unhealthy. Over the years, I've met countless families who refuse to accept the possibility of Huntington's Disease in their lives. They will not discuss it, even when both physical and mental symptoms make their protestations ridiculous.

At some point, refusing to acknowledge reality may be problematic in areas such as relationships, family planning, career and investment choices, and insurance issues. Accepting the possible existence of HD doesn't necessarily mean having to test for the gene, but it does mean learning as much as possible about the disease and planning for a possibly uncertain future.

Natalie didn't have to wear her father's briefs more than once or twice before she could sleep without fear of terrifying nocturnal visions. For Natalie, wearing her daddy's underpants—and more importantly, having faith in her daddy's promise—helped her to overcome her fears, and her nightmares stopped. But for people who persist in denying the possibility of HD, who refuse to recognize its symptoms, the nightmares may be only beginning. Real-life monsters just don't go away unless they are squarely faced and dealt with realistically. That happens only when the blinders—in Natalie's case, daddy's underpants—are purposely removed.

How about you? Are you or someone you love still wearing daddy's underpants?

Overkill

Do not anticipate trouble, or worry about what may never happen. Keep in the sunlight.

—BENJAMIN FRANKLIN

My sister, Diane, and I were on the phone recently. As happens more often than not, we began to swap stories.

"Carmen, I believe our neighbors used to wait 'till the sun went down, make their popcorn, sit on their porches, and wait for the show to begin."

"What neighbors? What house?" I asked.

"The one in Houston where Patricia and I lived before we both got married," she answered. "Everything that could go wrong, did go wrong. Even things that shouldn't have gone wrong, went wrong."

Since the same thing happens to me, I understood. Maybe it's genetic.

"So tell me what happened that particular time," I urged, egging her on.

One night, Diane, Patricia, and Diane's young son, Mario, slept peacefully in their little house. A few hours after settling down, Diane woke to a noise somewhere in the hushed night. At first it was barely perceptible but a noise none-the-less.

It seemed to come from the kitchen, and Diane held her breath as her heart began to beat wildly. The dull, barely discernable rustle turned into a scraping sound, like things being gently moved. Suddenly, the peaceful night was sinister, and Diane knew that someone, an intruder, was inside their home.

She listened for a bit, then crept silently into the adjacent bedrooms to alert the others to the danger. She cautioned them to be quiet as they tiptoed back to Diane's room. Back in her bedroom, after she'd grabbed the phone which had a long cord, the three stout-hearted Leals ensconced themselves in her bathroom. Once there, the door slightly ajar to keep track of the invader's movements, Diane called our other sister, Debbie, and her husband, Willie.

"Willie," she whispered, "there's a burglar in the house. Can you come over? Please? He's making a lot of noise in the kitchen."

Willie, ever calm, assured his frightened sister-in-law that not only would he come, he'd also call his friend, Paul, who lived less than a mile away. Comforted, Diane hung up. The three Leals huddled together, waiting for the worst. Still, with the bathroom door slightly ajar, they could hear every sound from the kitchen. The tension mounted.

After what seemed a long enough interval, Diane peeked out the bedroom door. The house filled with light. What on earth was going on! Worried that the intruder would attack, Diane kept her head low as she stealthily made her way from the bedroom to the front door.

The headlights of two patrol cars, complete with two officers with each car, nearly blinded her. Bringing up the rear were Willie and Paul... with rifles—long, menacing rifles, cocked and ready to kill! She stepped aside to let the entourage in and scurried back to the bedroom to wait while the police, Willie, and Paul faced whoever had invaded her home. She quickly told Patricia and Mario as the six men entered the kitchen, guns drawn. Silence. Then… laughter. They were laughing!

The three hostages, figuring there couldn't be that much danger if people were laughing, abandoned their hiding place. The six men, now relaxed with their guns holstered or propped against the wall, stood around the pantry. Laughing.

"We got your burglar," laughed Willie. The others chimed in as they stepped back to reveal the "burglar." There, still making noise, stood a mouse, a teeny, gray mouse. Six grown men with guns, four of them on salary, rushed out in the middle of the night to protect two damsels in distress from a mouse.

Diane doesn't remember exactly what happened to the mouse. Mario thinks they let him run outside. Someone mentioned a bag, a trip to the driveway, and tires. Well, you get the picture. What Diane does remember is the absolute heart-pounding terror she experienced when she first heard the middle-of-the-night kitchen noises.

Now it goes without saying that having a mouse in the kitchen comes nowhere near having HD or any other chronic or terminal disease. But it's the fear that's the issue, not the depth of its cause.

I'd wager some of you felt a fear not too dissimilar to my sister's panic when you first heard the words *Huntington's Disease*. That's understandable, given all this disease entails. Sometimes, though, we make things worse by playing the "what if" game.

What if, for example, violence happens? What if, before the driving stops, there's a fatal car wreck? What if a nursing home is the only answer?

Sometimes, we project the worst possible scenario. Not every person with Huntington's gets violent. Some people willingly give up driving, and many, many people are able to stay at home until the end. And Diane's burglar was really… only a mouse.

Just as in Diane's story, there is a place for caution. She didn't run into the kitchen armed with her son's baseball bat. That would have been foolhardy. Learning all you can about the stages of the disease, becoming active in support groups, both online and off, attending conventions, and reading all you can find, are all appropriate actions. Playing the "what if" game helps no one and can—and usually does—make things worse.

I wish I knew with certainty none of you were at risk, nor any of your children, or grandchildren will test positive. Wouldn't it be great if everyone who did inherit the gene would have late onset and mild symptoms? I can't predict the future and neither can you. But you can remember the mouse.

Years later, after they each married and moved away, my sisters both experienced what they had feared that night—a break in. While they were cautious, I'd like to think they remembered the mouse and didn't expect the worse. I also hope that as you deal with all that Huntington's is, you remember this: Your worst fears might never be realized.

Lessons from a Grouch

You must look into people, as well as at them.

—LORD CHESTERFIELD

"She can't sit here!"

Oh no, Cecilia was at it again. Was there anyone she liked in the entire nursing home? She really tried my patience. In fact, she actually made me reconsider how I was spending my time.

For the last six months I'd been doing a church service at Dave's nursing home. Even though I knew they, too, needed some sort of religious services, Cecilia gave me good reason to question if I was the person to fill that need.

"I said, no! I hate her," bellowed this geriatric complainer.

Cecilia never had visitors, and after only one week, I knew why. She was just plain nasty to most people, and she had long since lost her tact gene.

That day, after listening to her insult many people, I knew exactly what I would talk about: New Year's resolutions. No one is ever too old to change, I decided. This would be a great opportunity to let Cecilia know her behavior was not only rude and hurtful, it was also not pleasing to God.

After my opening song, I began to speak on my theme. I pulled together stories and music and was doing what I felt was a wonderful job.

As I reached to put a new accompaniment track into the cassette player, she interrupted me again.

"How much do those tapes cost?"

Trying to keep my patience, I told Cecilia they ranged anywhere from five to eight dollars.

"Each? That's a lot of money," she exclaimed. "How many do you have?"

"Well, that *is* a lot of money, and I have over 200. But I've been collecting them for many years, and I use them in my ministry."

"You need to learn to play the piano and stop buying tapes. Then you can spend your money on a pair of shoes. Those are ugly."

This was ridiculous. Her comment made me even more determined to give my message. She certainly needed to hear it. "My resolution," I said, in a somewhat self-righteous tone, "is to be more Christ-like and to draw closer to God."

I patted myself on the back so hard my arm nearly broke. After all, I was great at coming up with resolutions for my elders. Surely that covered anything anyone in the room would do in the new year, even Cecilia.

"No it's not."

Much beleaguered, I sighed heavily and said, "Excuse me? Cecilia, how can you tell me what my resolution is? It's my life, not yours."

Disregarding my obvious anger, Cecilia stared at me, looked around the room to make sure she had an audience, and made her proclamation.

"No. You need to say, 'My resolution is to lose weight.' You know why? You're too fat!"

My first inclination was to walk out and never come back. I just couldn't believe this obnoxious woman.

Maybe God did hear my resolution that afternoon because I did something totally opposite to what I wanted to do. I laughed. As I laughed, those in the room who could understand began to laugh. We laughed until we cried and laughed some more.

I realized I was taking all this way too seriously. Cecilia was right. I did need to lose weight and, no doubt, doing so would make me more Christ-like.

That was the beginning of the new Cecilia. While she still snapped at people now and then, she also smiled more and yelled less. She began to let me into her world with stories that helped me understand her anger and loneliness.

A few months later, Cecilia passed away in her sleep. Yes, she'd often been nasty and argumentative, but she had also helped me remember an important fact. Before ever needing twenty-four-hour care, people in nursing homes once had full, rich lives. She also helped me to laugh at myself. I'm a better person because of Cecilia.

Be Prepared

The best laid schemes o' mice an men go oft awry.

—ROBERT BURNS

Such a long list. And, according to the Peace Corps office, everything essential. I'd wanted to be a volunteer since the eighth grade, and now, in less than two weeks, I'd be on a plane to Atlanta.

Then, after being sworn in as a volunteer, my group of twenty-three would continue to New York's JFK airport and on to Abidjan, Ivory Coast. A quick flight to Bamako, Mali, and we'd spend our first night in Africa.

Between the going away parties and working, I'd spent every free moment shopping. The list had included not only clothing and shoes, but also a wide variety of personal items. It seemed impossible to think that all I needed in the middle of nowhere could fit into one checked bag and one carry-on.

Some suggested items weren't found in Mali, they said. These absolutely "must haves" included supplies for that "special" time of the month. With not a little embarrassment, I bought a two-year supply of the most compact-sized female products ever made.

As these were *so* important, I packed them into my carry-on duffle bag. Along with the tampons, I packed such things as a Tupperware pastry set and a few bottles of Avon

Skin So Soft, the best mosquito repellent made, intentionally or otherwise. I also tucked in aspirin, contact lens solution, and other essentials.

Fully packed and wondering if I'd made the right decision, I set off for an experience of a lifetime. The first leg of my journey from Kansas City ended with two days at one of the luxurious Peachtree hotels in downtown Atlanta. If you're from that bastion of southern society, or even if you've just visited, you know what I mean.

After who-knows-how-many vaccinations, and after taking the Peace Corps oath, we continued leg after leg until finally, over twenty-four hours later, we reached Mali's capital city, Bamako. Believe it or not, there really is a Timbuktu, and Bamako was just a bush taxi or boat ride away.

Twenty-three exhausted world travelers waited at the carousel. And waited, and waited. Welcome to Mali—no luggage. Not today, tomorrow, or ever. Though we'd been told what to bring for our two-year sojourn, we hadn't been told the unhappy fact that baggage theft in that part of the world is more common than not.

Almost too sleep-deprived to care, we walked into the furnace-like heat and followed our guides to the transportation. At least, I realized, I have what's in my carry-on, including my tampons.

After dinner, we had no choice but to disrobe and throw our clothes into the laundry so we'd have clean clothes for the next day. The blue denim skirt and yellow checked blouse were now my only American clothing. Again, I was relieved that, at least, I had my feminine supplies.

Following our first African breakfast, including tropical fruits, baguettes, and café au lait, one of the locals took us through the open-air market, showing us where to buy replacement clothing and anything else that had been in our lost luggage. Then we made one last stop before returning to the training center. The Super Marché, or supermarket, was about the size of an American convenience store. Canned milk, matches, toothpaste, and other common products from France lined the shelves. Making a mental inventory during my sweeping glance, I stopped short at the third wall. There, for anyone with enough francs, were boxes and boxes of tampons. I don't mean a dozen or so, I mean shelf after shelf of them!

I realized that, instead of bringing something in my carry-on I might need now that my luggage was gone, I had taken up over half the precious space with something apparently abundant in Mali. Oh well, I rationalized, ever the positive thinker, at least I had them and wouldn't have to spend any of my meager salary buying them.

Irony of ironies. Whether it was the water, the weather, or something else, I never had occasion to use even one of my precious tampons! Month after month I waited, and month after month nothing happened. On that last day, when I left Mali, I placed my supply in a basket and left them for the next volunteer. I sure hope a female moved in.

Remember the *Skin So Soft*? In another amazing turn of events, I developed an immunity to mosquitoes. The first six weeks, I was a mosquito buffet so often that huge welts swelled up. At first I thought it was a sun allergy, but eventually I realized that they were bites. Evidently, as a result, I am now virtually immune to whatever makes mosquito bites sting. And there I was with bottles and bottles of repellent. (At least my skin was silky-soft and hydrated.)

If you face Huntington's Disease, there are so many issues to deal with. Insurance, long term costs, social security, and that's only the beginning. Just as I planned on what to bring to Africa, we all need to plan as best we can for the future. But as I learned then, sometimes our best plans go awry—for any number of reasons. That's another lesson I learned: to have a "Plan B," or even a "Plan X, Y, or Z" on back-up. And while you're reworking your plans, make sure to laugh.

Laughter

---

*You grow up the day you have your first
real laugh—at yourself.*

—ETHEL BARRYMORE

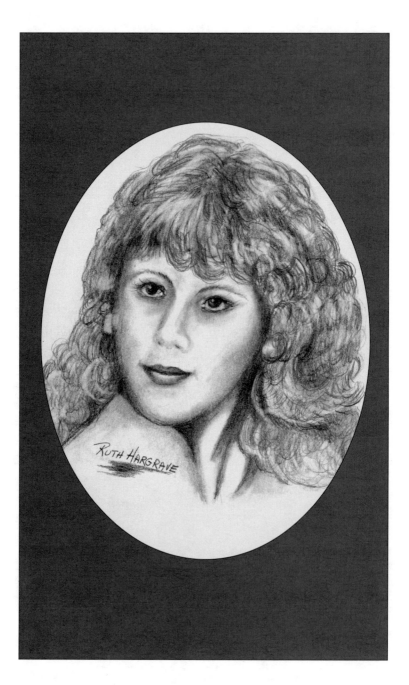

The Girl with the Talking Eyes

One of the most wonderful things in nature is a glance of the eye; it transcends speech; it is the bodily symbol of identity.

—RALPH WALDO EMERSON

Kimberly Darlene Brown touched many people in her too-short life. The day of the visitation at the funeral home, people came to pay their respects one last time. They came because Kim had had that indefinable something that drew people to her.

Flowers came from a school she hadn't attended in eight years. People who had spent only one day with her came, former teachers, counselors, hospice nurses, and social workers were there, right along with her young friends. Even all of her brother's friends and their spouses stood in line to say good-bye.

Twenty-four years earlier, on June 11, 1974 in Groton, Connecticut, Paul and Cheryl Brown greeted their precious Kim. Even big brother, Wes, was excited. The Brown's precious new bundle was a healthy, ten-pound baby who grew quickly, developing normally throughout childhood.

For most of Kim's life, the Brown's lived near a section of an interstate highway that, hard as it is to believe, people used as dumping grounds for troublesome pets. Stray dogs and cats constantly roamed the neighborhood, foraging in the garbage cans, which drove Kim's father crazy.

The poor dogs eventually moved on, until one day when Kim was five. One little dog refused to understand that "git" was meant for her, too. She cringed, but she wasn't about to leave. Cheryl didn't have to wonder for long why this particular canine was so stubborn. One day she saw Kim feeding the scavenger on the sly.

"Kim, you must not feed the dog," said Cheryl, staring at the defiant little girl. "You're just making it harder for everyone. When your dad gets tired of all the mess this dog is making, he'll do what is necessary to get rid of her.

The next morning, Kim and Cheryl heard Paul yelling. Peering out the window, the two saw him standing in a yard full of garbage, flailing his arms and shouting at the dog. "You git! Now!" The louder Paul yelled, the firmer the dog stood her ground. She wasn't going anywhere.

Finally, in a rage, Paul kicked the dog. In a flash, Kim hurtled out the door into the yard and ran straight to her dad, kicking him in the shins as hard as her little feet could kick. "I held my breath as she placed her hands on her hips," said Cheryl, "looking all the world like Shirley Temple fighting a crusade."

"You are not supposed to kick animals," shouted the little blond tornado. "How do you like someone kicking you?"

While Cheryl could support Kim's feelings, she held her breath, anticipating Paul's reaction. Paul stared down at his little daughter and did the unexpected—he laughed. Kim's head jerked up in surprise, and she looked into his eyes.

Cheryl and Paul knew their little Kim was a spunky child who didn't hold back when it came to championing the "underdog." They saw Kim's productive attitude toward this helpless, homeless animal as a good sign; Kim had the right kind of "stuff."

Always happy and sociable, Kim couldn't wait to start school. As bright as she was though, there were learning problems. At age eleven, she was finally diagnosed as dyslexic. She attended a special school for dyslexic children. That "stuff" carried her through some difficult years.

Kim took much teasing because she moved slowly and was "different" from other kids. One February, Cheryl remembers Kim receiving a notice for a semi-formal school dance. "She was so excited," says Cheryl. "She was going, even if she had to go alone. She was no different from any other girl her age, and my heart broke for what I knew could happen."

Like other girls, Kim had crushes on the cute, popular guys; guys who wouldn't give her a first glance, much less a second. So, just as Cheryl feared, no one asked Kim to the dance.

"Kim was true to her word," Cheryl explained. "If no one wanted to go with her, too bad. She'd go alone. And that's exactly what she did."

When Cheryl dropped Kim at the gym, she looked gorgeous. Any mother would be proud of such a beautiful daughter. Nestled with that pride, though, was worry—worry that when she came back to pick her up after the dance, she would find a very dejected young lady.

"I was out there in the parking lot at the agreed-upon time, practicing my smiles, hugs, and 'Oh well' speech." Before long, Kim came out of the door on the arm of a young man, who, before helping her into the car, gently kissed her good night.

"Kim was glowing," Cheryl remembers with delight. "Introducing himself, the young man waved to me and told me I had a beautiful daughter. He smiled at her and thanked her for a wonderful evening. We said goodnight and left."

As cliché as it sounds, Kim really was in "seventh heaven." The young man, who didn't attend the same school, had come that evening with friends. He danced not only the first dance with Kim, but every dance! When they weren't dancing, they sat and talked, and he attended to her refreshments as a gentleman should.

"Best of all, he treated her as special as she was. I knew she was special, but so was he. Kim never saw him again after that night."

Every woman deserves a knight in shining armor at some time in her life. Cheryl often thanks God for that knight. It took a remarkable young man to dance every dance, not with the belle of the ball, but with the one most likely to be a wallflower. I'm sure he's still a remarkable man. In one short night, he made an enormous impact on Kim's self-esteem.

When she was sixteen, Kim tested back into the public school system under the "educable mentally-handicapped program." Later that year, she was diagnosed with Juvenile Huntington's Disease and entered the physically disabled program at school.

Kim didn't let the changes get her down. With her winning personality, she was the manager of the band flag corps in a specially created position. She also sang in the choir one year, attended all the school football games and many of the social functions, including the senior prom.

His name was Kevin, and even though he was a year younger, Kevin and Kim ate lunch together just about every day. They were in love. Kevin had cerebral palsy, but he made her cards and wrote her love notes on his computer. Kevin even took extra credits in summer school so that he could graduate with her.

Then, in their senior year, Kevin invited Kim to the prom. Because of his disability, Kevin was unable to drive. So his health-care attendant, along with his girl-friend, agreed to drive the young couple and stay to give any needed help.

The wait for the van was interminable. When it did arrive, Kevin insisted on being taken inside to present Kim with her corsage. Cheryl pinned it on as Kevin grinned and beamed.

What a special evening it was! Following their seafood buffet dinner, this special couple entered the enchanted world of the senior prom. Kevin and Kim danced, he in the wheelchair, she on her feet, holding his hands as she moved to the music. After dancing and enjoying an evening with their friends, Kim's Prince Charming escorted her home in his mother's van, which doubled as Kim's pumpkin carriage.

"Kim glowed for days," remembers Cheryl. "For days, Kevin repeated the same phrase, but his mother couldn't understand his garbled speech. A few days later, I got a call from Kevin's mom wanting Kim to know what Kevin had been saying. 'Mom, she was gorgeous!'" Kim insisted she was in love with Kevin until the day she died.

Kim graduated from high school in the spring of 1994. Then, in February of 1995, she was hospitalized for the first time with complications caused by JHD. The seizures she suffered were to mark the beginning of the end for Kim and, after that, she never walked again. Over the next three years, this young woman with the indomitable spirit was moved from wheelchair to hospital bed.

"People often told me Kim had the most expressive face they had ever seen," shares Cheryl. "When they came to know her better, they realized that it was her eyes. They were big, round, and blue, with long thick lashes."

Remembering those eyes, Cheryl continues, "From the time Kim was very young, her eyes spoke volumes. When she was little, she couldn't lie. Not that she didn't try, her eyes just told on her. All of her life they reflected her feelings: anticipation, anger, hurt, sadness, fear, worry, and, best of all—sheer joy. When she was happy, those eyes, coupled with that wonderful smile, absolutely changed her whole appearance."

Even when she was ill and too weak to speak, her eyes still spoke, telling her loving family all they needed know. As the parish priest so aptly stated, "There is grace behind those eyes."

At home, surrounded by those she loved, Kim closed her eyes one day and could not open them, and Cheryl knew Kim would be leaving them soon. She passed away the next morning, December 1, 1998.

Yes, people came to say goodbye to Kim that last day. Of course they came to support her family, but mostly they came for an exceptional young woman with a beautiful smile, a great sense of humor, and talking eyes.

Musical Memories

After silence, that which comes nearest to expressing the
inexpressible is music.

—ALDOUS HUXLEY

"Music is the way our memories sing to us across time." This quote by Lance Morrow is especially appropriate for the Brown family.

On the second anniversary of her daughter's death, Cheryl Brown planned to keep herself busy. Her agenda for the day: a trip to the cemetery to visit Kim, then on to the bank and the mall. But it wasn't to be.

"I wasn't able to do any of those things. I felt a bit down."

Before her son, Wes, left for work that morning, Cheryl remembers him calling out, "Mom, I want you to listen to this today. I made it for you."

Curious about his creation, Cheryl placed the compact disc into the player and began to listen to her memories.

"As I listened to the music, I cried and I laughed. Wes had compiled a collection of songs important because Kimberly was part of our lives."

"I will always keep the CD," Cheryl says. "But the real treasure is the young man. Wes was a wonderful brother. He has feeling and depth beyond the surface, and he is my son."

What do you say to your mother to take away the loss she will feel and relive each anniversary? There aren't enough words to share the emotion of loss. Leo Tolstoy says, "Music is the shorthand of emotion."

Here is a list of the "shorthand" one special young man compiled for his mother. I agree that Cheryl's son does have feeling and depth and a whole lot more. I've included Cheryl's comments about why some of the songs are special.

"Angel Flying too Close to the Ground," by Willie Nelson

"Beautiful, Beautiful, Beautiful Boy," by John Lennon, lyrics by Yoko Ono

"I Love You a Bushel and a Peck," by Frank Loesser

"I Love to See You Smile," by Randy Newman

"I Am Your Angel," by R. Kelley

"You Picked a Fine Time to Leave Me, Lucille," by Kenny Nelson *(or, as little Kimi used to sing, "You Picked a Fine Time to Leave Me to Sears")*

"Mrs. Brown, You've Got a Lovely Daughter," by Herman's Hermits *(We told her the song was about her.)*

"The Never Ending Story," by Georgio Moroder, lyrics by Keith Forsey *(one of her favorite movies)*

"Stand By Me," by Ben E. King, Jerry Leiber, and Mike Stoller *(This was her all-time-favorite movie. She had the dialogue memorized.)*

"The Dance," by Tony Arata *(her favorite country singer and her favorite song)*

"Together Again," by Janet Jackson

"True Colors," by Tom Kelly, Billy Steinberg

"An Uncloudy Day," by Willie Nelson/Bobbie Nelson

"Wind Beneath My Wings," by Larry Henley and Jeff Silbar

He Who Laughs, Lasts

*Let us be of good cheer, remembering that the misfortunes
hardest to bear are those which never happen.*

—JAMES RUSSELL LOWELL

At the age of eighteen, I developed a goiter and underwent major thyroid surgery. My parathyroid, which controls calcium, required removal as well. I can't be sure whether or not that was the reason, but since that April surgery, I've been a nail biter.

I've never been particularly concerned about my short nails, so I have never exercised any self-discipline to curtail what really is only a bad habit. Well, a couple of weeks ago, I claimed a prize package that I won in a random drawing from a furniture store.

My prize, including a facial, hair style, manicure, and pedicure, seemed almost laughable; I don't wear make up, and I have no nails to speak of. But since I needed a new press and book photo anyway, I decided to get glamorous before the photo session.

After my manicure, I held to my resolve not to bite my nails. After a time, though, I needed to file them and reapply some new polish, as the original stuff had become old and chipped. Of course, I don't own anything like a file or nail polish, so on my way to see Dave one day, I went shopping. I am only marginally better at shopping than I am at manicuring, but I bought a file, polish remover, clear nail polish, those little cuticle stick things, and cotton balls. Talk about a stranger in a foreign land!

Because I could no longer transfer Dave by myself, we stopped going to the movies and other almost-daily outings. Instead, we now spend our time in the nursing home or, on nice days, in the garden. I arrange my days and visits around his favorite show, "The Price is Right." We've fallen into a nice routine while we watch the contestants "Come on down."

On this particular day, I settled him in his Broda chair and found seating for myself. I pulled up the bedside table on wheels and took out my manicure supplies. Pouring remover onto the little cotton ball, I began taking off the old nail polish while watching the show.

"You look good today, Dave," I cheerfully commented as I moved the cotton ball over each nail. I continued chatting about this and that, all the while glancing at the screen.

All of a sudden I looked up, and Dave was staring at my nails and laughing! Soundlessly laughing.

"You find this amusing, do you?"

From the remover to the polish, with the filing, cuticles, and buffing in between, Dave laughed. He continued laughing from the first contestant all the way to the first showcase showdown, stopping only after I'd finished my nails.

People often ask, "Does Dave know what's going on?" My answer is a resounding, "Yes!"

People with Huntington's Disease may not be able to express themselves as they once could, but their memories are intact. Dave has always had a great sense of humor. It might have been hidden for a time until the medications worked their "magic," but he knows what's going on.

I have two goals. Seeing Dave laugh fills us both with joy. I want to experience that joy whenever I'm with him. I am also determined to grow these nails, but I get the impression Dave doesn't believe I will succeed and, contrary as always, I'm determined to prove him wrong. The last laugh will be mine!

Proof Positive

Each of us is an accumulation of our memories.

—ALAN LOY MCGINNIS

Today I went to see Dave at the nursing home. As is becoming our tradition, we settled down to watch "The Price is Right." During one segment, the contestants were trying to get up on stage by guessing the correct price of the baby furniture being featured.

I glanced at Dave and noticed his smile as he stared intently at the screen.

"You had babies, didn't you, Dave?" I asked.

He smiled—a huge grin—but remained silent. Of course, that didn't surprise me since neither I, nor anyone else, had heard him speak a word in over a year. Still, as I firmly believe it helps both of us, I always talk to him and ask questions, in an attempt to help him enjoy life as much as possible.

"What are their names?" I questioned.

In easily understood words, Dave answered, "Andy and Jessica."

"What?" I nearly shrieked when I heard those three words come from him with such little effort. "You can talk! Dave, why do you never talk to me? What else can you say?"

With an almost smug look on his lean face, he calmly answered with one word: "Everything."

The entire exchange took place amidst his laughter and my confusion. For over a year, I'd struggled with his inability to talk. Why, I'd told everyone he couldn't talk. Yet, here he was answering my questions.

"What's your dad's name?" I quizzed.

"Charlie," he responded on cue.

"How about your brother's name?"

"Fred."

This one-word answer shocked me. Fred was his brother who had died of crib death over forty-five years ago, and yet Dave remembered.

After I got over my surprise, I continued. "Who's your other brother?"

"Daryl."

Okay, four for four. Let's do one more, I thought.

"What's your ex-wife's name?"

Prepared to hear his ex's given name, Dave threw me another curveball.

Every shred of humor left Dave's face and eyes. As clearly as you or I, he responded with a word that sounded very similar to "Witch!"

I laughed so hard I fell off the chair. Then he laughed that soundless laugh of his. It was delightfully funny.

"No Dave," I finally corrected after I could breathe again, "You know her name."

From Dave's description of his previous marriage, his word choice sounded appropriate to me. The few times I'd talked to her over the phone, she certainly lived up to that label. Still, it seemed mean, so I asked him once again. "So, what's her name?"

"Witch," he responded with finality.

After our family-tree exchange, Dave clammed up and

focused his attention on Bob Barker's beauties prancing around in high heels and swim suits, showing off a motor boat. Try as I would, and believe me, I tried, Dave would not utter one more sound, let alone word.

One thing I've learned about Huntington's Disease is that it's unpredictable. Just when you think you've figured it out, something happens and you start all over again, trying to understand. I've mentioned in talks and chat rooms that people with HD retain their memories and their personality, it's just hard to see that most days.

The next time you wonder at the truth of those comments, I suggest you remember Dave. He's proof positive.

The Infamous African Toilet Story

A man without mirth is like a wagon without springs. He is jolted disagreeably by every pebble in the road.

—ANONYMOUS

Would the clenched muscles of my sore backside ever relax? A hot shower sounded like a slice of heaven, however the chances of that happening ranged from zero to none.

Experiencing West Africa felt like living in the pages of a *National Geographic* magazine. Definitely fascinating. But after weeks of traveling by bush taxi, I wanted comfort.

A bush taxi is the most readily available and affordable method of transportation in West Africa. Whether in Mali, home base for my two-year Peace Corps stint, or other countries I visited such as Senegal, Niger, Togo, or Ivory Coast, bush taxis rarely varied.

They start with a pickup truck, preferably one without shock absorbers. This gives the rider a true, jaw-clenching, bone-jolting experience. By law, a bush taxi cannot be new, and by definition, the tires must be as bald as possible. This increases the odds of breaking down in the middle of the desert or some other barren terrain. To further enhance the true African bush-taxi experience, passengers sit on hard planks of wood fashioned into benches, jammed into the bed of the truck. Did I mention the wood is not sanded?

This makes for a fun, post-travel activity called, "pulling splinters out of one's rear."

No bush-taxi trip is authentic without a minimum of fifteen people crammed into a space typically suitable for no more than eight. Of course that doesn't include the chickens and the occasional goat who get to ride for free.

Bush taxis operate on the "that depends" schedule. When do they leave? That depends on when enough people have paid and are ready to leave. How much is the ride? That depends on how many people are willing to go and, in large part, your fluency in the native language. The less fluent, the higher the price. When will we arrive? That depends on how often we break down, if and when tires, gasoline, or spare parts are found, and how many potty-breaks we take.

Which brings us to the part most likely to strike terror in the hearts of female travelers, especially *tubobs*, or foreigners. Not surprisingly, when traversing regions such as those in West Africa, you'll find few Howard Johnson's, fast-food restaurants, or filling stations—let alone bathrooms. When the bush taxi stops, everyone files out to stretch their legs, whether nature is calling or not. When nature does call, choose a spot, any spot. Since my African travels, I have lost any modesty I ever possessed. With few trees and no buildings—and usually as the lone and always sole, foreign female—I became the focal point of every break.

After more than twelve hours of travel, you can imagine my joy at pulling into the taxi station in Ouagadougou, Upper Volta, now known as Ouagadougou, Burkina Faso.

Like most cities, Ouagadougou boasts a Grand Marche, or open market, and the taxi station sits next door.

As we pulled into the station that evening, I saw vultures feasting on the remains of the market meat. I couldn't tell for sure if those vultures wcrc enjoying beef, lamb, goat, rat, or cat carcass, since Africa is the land of the "don't ask, don't tell" cuisine.

Spying a hotel, we got our luggage, such as it was, and headed off towards a soft bed. Upon seeing the hanging sign above the door, I burst out laughing. To this day, I'd love to know the story behind the name "Hotel California!"

The Hotel California had none of the comforts of California, including an elevator. We trudged upstairs to the fifth floor, wondering if our cramped feet and legs would support us all the way. They did, but just barely.

The less-than-fresh linen covering the sway-back bed didn't deter me for a second. I unceremoniously threw myself down, relieved not to be on a wooden plank in a jostling truck. My equally weary future husband quickly followed suit, and we both fell into a deep sleep.

Nature does have a way of calling, and that's exactly what happened a few hours later. Adjusting my eyes to the blackness, I panned the room for a light switch or lamp. Failing to find one, I got up and gingerly made my way across the room, hoping to avoid contact with uninvited guests of the rodent or insect variety. As my eyes grew accustomed to the dark, I realized that what I sought did not exist. No toilet. No bidet.

Things were getting serious, so I looked for something, anything, to use as a receptacle. Nothing. No cup. No glass. No can. Nothing even remotely able to hold the threatening liquid.

"Honey, wake up," I urged, as I shook Nick's shoulder once I got back to bed. "I need to go to the bathroom."

I was sure Nick wondered why I felt the need to wake *him* for such an announcement, so I clarified my need. "Nick. There's no toilet here and no bathroom on this floor. Would you walk me downstairs so I can use the bathroom down there?"

"I'm tired. Go downstairs and leave me alone," answered this paragon of chivalry.

I couldn't believe what I was hearing. Go downstairs by myself? With no electricity, I might step on tarantulas, geckos, or worse still, some small animal waiting to pounce. No way was I going by myself.

I could either go in the bed—but somehow that didn't seem like the best option—or I could do something else. My eyes, now adjusted to the darkened room, spied a sink in the corner. As my bladder grew more uncomfortable, a plan began to form.

Now, I'm what many call a "full-figured girl," and have been, since I came out of my mother's womb, a size sixteen. All right, I exaggerate, but I definitely take after my father's side of the family. Still, desperation calls for imagination, so I made my way to the corner, hoisted myself to near sitting position over the sink, somehow balanced myself, and opened my bladder. At least I tried to open it. Before I could accomplish my goal, I felt the sink move and heard an ominous groaning sound. The sink crashed off the wall, hitting me on the calves and knocking me to the floor.

"Nick," I cried, rushing to the bed. "Please, get up! There's water everywhere and we need to leave. Now!"

"What did you do?" yelled Nick, groggy yet coherent.

Of course one look at lake Hotel California persuaded Sir Gallant to escort me to the lobby—with our luggage.

Once outside the hotel, we went to the marché where we sat and waited for the first bush taxi anywhere. I still feel guilty leaving such a mess and breaking the sink, but what could I do?

At the station, needing to answer that yet unanswered call of nature, I did what *Nike* intended as a slogan for something completely different from my situation; I just did it.

We huddled together, hoping no one from the police or hotel would arrive on the scene to arrest us. If they came, hopefully it would be after we were on the next taxi to Benin. Not the best choice since we ended up in jail. That's another story for another book.

Try as I might, I couldn't find a lesson in this anecdote related to HD. I hope the story made you laugh though, because when dealing with Huntington's Disease, we all need to laugh—often, as much as possible.

Patience

The greatest prayer is patience.

—GAUTAMA BUDDA

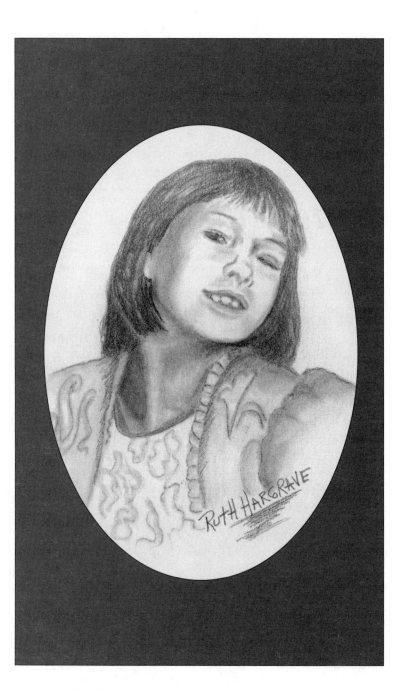

Little Miss Sunshine

The poor give us much more than we give them. They're such strong people, living day to day with no food and they never curse, never complain. We don't have to give them pity or sympathy. We have so much to learn from them.

—MOTHER TERESA

Devastating as Huntington's Disease is, I think there's something even worse: Juvenile Huntington's Disease. There's something about children who have barely begun to live being stricken with something we cannot fix.

Shannon was born to Shayne and Patricia Meyers on October 27, 1988. She was a normal, six-pound baby girl who captured the hearts of everyone she met. Until she was three, Shannon was advanced in everything. She walked early, and talked early, and even changed her own clothes because she wanted to wear what she wanted to wear.

When Shannon was three, her parents noticed that her speech was slurred. A speech evaluation resulted in a recommendation for a complete developmental evaluation. What with Shayne's recent diagnosis of Huntington's Disease, this was cause for great concern.

"She's too young," her parents kept saying. "This is impossible."

They were stunned. After Shayne was diagnosed, he and Pat, like most parents at the beginning of this topsy-turvy journey with HD, thought first of Shannon. Had she, too, inherited the gene? But doctors reassured them. Huntington's was an adult-only disease, and they'd shelved their concerns for her, at least until she was older.

When they discovered after more research that there *was* a juvenile form of the disease, they were devastated. But their depression lifted after the evaluation was done with no signs of Juvenile Huntington's Disease. The doctors recommended, and Shannon received, physical therapy.

For about two years, everything seemed fine. When Shannon started falling more, denial made it easier to believe she was simply clumsy. But the school wanted a complete evaluation done, even though Shannon, a bright girl, did well in school. The physical "things" were just not right.

Then, when Shannon was eight years old, there was a dramatic personality change. The smiling, loving Shannon was gone, and in her place was an angry little girl, almost impossible to put up with.

The neurologist saw no signs of Juvenile Huntington's Disease, but he did prescribe Ritalin. He also recommended that she be tested for Juvenile Huntington's Disease. Partly because they knew there wasn't a cure, and partly to spare themselves, they decided not to test. How could they tell their beautiful, eight-year-old daughter that she might have a disease they couldn't fix? Some things you can't deal with. This was one of those things: a doctor telling them their daughter was going to die. So, life continued, pretty much the same.

After another year, through the falls, Shannon started getting worse. Things that had once come easily to her were now insurmountable. Shannon, who could dress herself at the age of three, now couldn't button a button, much less dress herself. Drinking from a straw became impossible. To go on denying her the test was no longer feasible.

Then the unthinkable finally became reality. On July 5, 1998, when she was nine years old, Shannon was diagnosed with Juvenile Huntington's Disease.

A lot has changed since that day in 1988 when Shannon entered the world, but not everything. She is still a bright and loving little girl. She still smiles all the time, and she still says, "I love you." She also still captures the hearts of everyone who meets her. Like many twelve-year-old girls, Shannon loves animals and rainbows. Her anger phase seems to be over, and everything she owns is yellow, matching her sunny personality.

For Pat, life is challenging; she has both a husband and a daughter to care for. "Once in awhile they will both have a good day and I just love it," says Pat. "They are rare though." Besides all the normal household chores, Pat feeds, bathes, and dresses Shannon, takes her for all her doctor's appointments, monitors her medication, and gets her to and from school one or two days a week on average.

Shayne still feeds himself, as long as the food is placed in front of him. It's hard, though. Both Shannon and her father have awkward sleeping schedules, so Pat naps when she can.

"Both my husband and Shannon are remarkable," explains Pat. "They do not ever complain about this disease, not even when they can't do something they used to do. Oh, they still have their obsessions and stubborn moods. They still get angry at times over minor things. Sometimes I don't even know what they're upset about, as neither can talk well. Despite all this, they simply don't complain about having this terrible disease."

Disappointment has become such a big part of Shannon's life. Juvenile Huntington's differs in many ways from the adult version. Seizures are commonplace in children, so Shannon is now on medication for them. Despite the medication, it seems every time something is planned, she has a seizure. On one occasion, Shannon was excited about going on a school field trip to see a play. She talked about it all evening, making sure her lunch was packed and her money and permission slip sent in.

After a good sleep, she was up and off to school, all smiles. About twenty minutes later, Pat got the dreaded seizure call.

"Shannon, honey. I'm so sorry you had a seizure and had to miss another field trip," comforted Pat.

"That's okay, Mom," said Shannon with a big smile. The missed field trip was never mentioned again.

When Shannon was first diagnosed, the first question Pat asked was, "God, how are we going to deal with this?" Although she doesn't know what will come next, she does know all she can do is live life one day at a time.

"It's Shannon's strength I draw off of when I'm down," remarks Pat. "If she and her father can lose so much and not complain, who am I to complain? That's how I get through the days that are really bad. With God's help," she continues, "and the love and support of many friends and family members, we will make life as pleasant and loving as possible for as long as she has. And we will pray for a cure."

Just Doing My Job

God helps them that help themselves.

—AUTHOR UNKNOWN

I'm a self-sufficient person who tends to find the proverbial glass half full instead of half empty. Suddenly, though, I felt half empty, running dangerously close to the red indicator mark. How could I continue alone?

Dave and I had left Hawaii, moving away from our friends, church, and support system. At the time, there seemed to be no alternative, but now I was wondering if welfare might have made more sense. I'd just have to demand home health care, even though I knew he didn't really qualify because he didn't need "skilled medical care."

Dave's doctor seemed to be a caring man, but knew only the textbook information about Huntington's Disease. Since there was no neurologist who accepted Medicaid in our area, the doctor and I had to learn all we could. Together, we would figure out the best way to make sure Dave got all the help he needed.

One day, after juggling resources to make sure I could afford Dave's food and medication, I took him to the doctor. Before that, I'd stood in line at the foodbank to ask for help feeding my children since our meager funds wouldn't stretch that month. That, combined with having a church pay for our utilities, would see us through the month at least.

83

One day at a doctor's appointment, readying myself for "battle," I took a deep breath before plunging in. "Doctor, is there any way we can get a home health aide for Dave? It's getting hard to do everything by myself."

I expected a yes or no. What I didn't expect was the answer I got. "I think Dave is doing worse than he should be because he's married to you."

"… Excuse me?"

"Yes. You're not handling this well, and he's picking up on that. I think you need counseling."

Counseling. I came in to get someone to help bathe and feed my husband only to be told I was not "handling it well." Who would handle a terminally ill husband, who needed practically everything done for him? Well? Was this man crazy?

When I could finally speak again, I did. "You're right," I answered with the most sarcasm I could muster. "You're absolutely right. I do need counseling. The problem is, I have no health insurance or money for counseling. But then, I'm sure that as I am so desperately in need of counseling, and as you are such a compassionate person, you'll be happy to pay for it."

Disregarding the look on his face, I shot off my other suggestions rapid-fire. "Oh, and Doctor, as long as you'll be watching my husband while I get counseling, could you clean the house? I really haven't had the time. Dave spills and falls and breaks things, and somehow, my house is always a mess. Why not do the laundry, too? Between Dave and my two sons, there's a never-ending pile of laundry that needs doing. While you're there anyway, could you cook dinner and help the children with their homework? I need the checkbook balanced and you might want to slip out and do some grocery shopping since we're running low on food."

Speechless, the doctor stared at me, probably thinking I was going to explode if I talked any faster. Before he thought of anything to say, I went in for the kill.

"And Doctor," I smiled sweetly. "I haven't had sex for a long, long time. Now, you're short, fat, and balding, so I'm not interested. But if you could find me someone to have sex with, I might not need counseling!"

Without a word, the doctor took his pad and wrote a prescription for a home health aide.

Things got better after I had some help. The aides the doctor ordered were covered by Medicare and helped me care for Dave.

Most caregivers of someone severely ill have problems such as I've mentioned in this story, yet others so seldom stop to realize these things. This episode I've shared here is only a drop in the proverbial bucket of usually unmentioned feelings. But those of you who have ever been a caregiver certainly understand how desperate I felt that day.

A talk I give at HD conferences is called, "We All Have a Job to Do." In this talk I discuss all the jobs involved in making sure loved ones get the care they need. I'm not suggesting that seeking outside help is something you *need* to do, but if you think it will help, by all means, go for it. Desperate times call for desperate measures. Hey, I was just doing my job.

"Bad Dog, Bad Dog!"

A dog is the only thing on this earth that loves you more than he loves himself.

—JOSH BILLINGS

The other day Dave and I were having a conversation. I talk with my mouth, and he answers with his huge brown eyes and sometimes a smile. We were watching TV and a commercial featuring a dog was aired. I reminded Dave about his boyhood pet, Eddie. Taking Dave's smile as a signal to continue, I launched into the topic of Brutus.

Brutus was as an engaging puppy. His big, brown puppy eyes just begged us to keep him. His champagne-colored fur, the color women pay fortunes to wear, was soft and silky.

Naturally, my children begged for the dog. "Can we keep him, Mom? We'll never be bad again. We'll take care of him ourselves. You won't even know he's here!" They spouted every excuse little boys can drum up in the space of three minutes. Each reason given by the boys was echoed by Dave, and he even added a few of his own.

Until then, these sons of mine hadn't been too sure about my fiancé, Dave. Ever since they'd met him, they'd been acting as a united hedge around Mom to protect her from this interloper. But now there a crack in their defenses, and the three banded together to persuade me to keep the dog.

Under the weight of their pleas, I finally crumbled and said yes. The boys, spurred on by the thrill of ownership, rocketed to get their puppy.

Brutus had a peaceful first night at our house. We didn't hear a peep from him. Half standard poodle and half golden retriever, he was 100 percent adorable.

Trouble began when Brutus ate my mother's white shoes, purchased especially for my wedding. A rush to the hardware store for white paint, along with a, "Bad dog, bad dog!" took care of both problems.

The fun really started after the wedding. It seemed no matter what we tried, we simply could not train him. To conquer the problem, the boys and Dave eagerly trotted Brutus off to obedience training each Wednesday.

As bright as this bundle of joy was, the minute he walked into our home, it became his territory. Brutus quickly discovered that, during the day, the house was his kingdom, and he was King Brutus. As we worked and studied, Brutus frolicked through his castle, ate shoes and other delectable belongings, devoured any food left in his sight, and generally wreaked havoc on his surroundings.

No matter what we tried, this dog was out of our control. The glass-topped coffee table near the window became a throne on which he sunned himself each day. One day, the throne crashed because of his ever-increasing weight, leaving shards of glass strewn across the floor. Brutus sat cowering, waiting for the phrase he'd so often heard: "Bad dog, bad dog!"

Then there was the day wind slammed the door shut and trapped him in our bedroom. He clawed his way out of the hollow-core door, leaving a two-foot, jagged hole in his wake.

Brutus, relentless in his quest for food, discovered an ability to open the refrigerator door. Oh, the glories of food that were his! As if he was doing something wonderful for me, Brutus carted his prizes to *my* side of the bed. He then proceeded to deposit chunks of food, doggie slobber, and other less-than-delightful presents onto my bedspread.

Each time I determined to call the pound, the children cried. They would do anything to keep their dog—pay for the damage, train him—"Please Mom, please!" They even tried using guilt to make their point. First it was Dad, now it's Brutus.

As my guilt increased, so did pressure to keep the dog. Meanwhile, the damage to my home continued and I despaired of ever reclaiming domestic peace and tranquility. When the broken door through which he escaped to roam the neighborhood was fixed, Brutus the Wonderdog found the window to be an alternative route. Never mind the glass and screen. Off he went on another exploration.

Finally, there came The Day. The lines had been drawn and Brutus had crossed them all. The damage, the dirt, the incessant barking, all contributed to the ultimatum. This dog must go. The tears coursed down their faces as my sons wailed in protest. I was the worst mother in the world. And all the time, as the battle raged, my husband silently sat with an accusing stare. Finally, exhausted, I promised I'd sleep on it and have a decision by morning.

The house grew quiet, and I turned to God to help with my dilemma. As if He were not fully aware of the situation, I pleaded my cause, stressing just how bad the situation had become with this eighty-pound terror. I justified my actions, convinced He would agree. But the peace I expected to have once I'd made a decision simply would not come. I tossed and turned until finally, I went into the living room to sit on the remainder of the sofa Brutus had ravaged.

As I sat, close to tears, I peered under the kitchen table. There was Brutus. His soft snores whistled through the silent house. I weighed my options as the indecision mounted. I cried out my anguish. I knew my sons would survive the loss of Brutus, but would I survive their anger and hurt?

My sons cleaned up after Brutus each time he made a mess. They offered up their allowance to pay for the damages, endured rainy nights to walk him, and listened to endless hours of complaints from neighbors after each barking rampage. To them, Brutus could do no wrong grave enough to merit being taken to the pound. They were even willing to plead his case to their mean-spirited, heartless mother. They had an unconditional love for their dog at which I marveled.

Thus, Brutus lived at our house until we moved to a new state 5,000 miles away. We didn't replace him after that, much to my sons' disappointment. With Huntington's Disease, I felt I had enough to deal with.

As Dave progressed while living at home, the damages to the house mounted. Drywall gave way to Dave's fist as poor balance forced him to catch himself before falling. Random movements while eating resulted in food splashed on walls and furniture. Carpets, floors, and bathrooms all took a beating.

I'd like to say I never lost my temper and wiped up each spill with a patient smile. I'd be lying if I told you I accepted each disaster, large or small, by giving Dave a hug. I can tell you, however, that Brutus made a lasting impression on me. Usually when I wanted to scream at Dave for yet another broken or dirtied item, I'd remember my sons' unconditional love for their pet. To them, their love for that dog was pure and worth everything in their lives. I found myself trying to emulate that unconditional love with Dave, and, more often than not, it worked.

"Unconditional" means, "without limitations or mitigating conditions" (*American Heritage Dictionary*). It also means having compassion when one wants to be anything but compassionate. That Dave doesn't behave exactly like the man I married doesn't matter. He's still my Dave and he is loved.

The dog catcher always said Brutus was a great dog, just not a city dog. In an ironic twist, when we moved, she asked if Brutus could live with her on nine acres with many other dogs. I'm sure he's having a great time and hearing, "Bad dog, bad dog!" a lot less often.

I hope he still misses us because we still miss him. Even Mom.

Bad Naked

Everything comes to him who hustles while he waits.

—THOMAS A. EDISON

It's amazing how the best of days can be sabotaged and turned into your worst nightmare.

One day a few summers ago, with the children visiting their father in Hawaii and Dave in bed, I could finally get some work done. Every time I tried to clean up one mess, Dave would make another. It's not that he intentionally tried to knock over dishes or smash his fist through the drywall when he fell. His increasingly bad balance and poor judgment turned my house into a disaster area.

With twenty-four ounces of chocolate *Boost* in his tummy and another twelve ounces of water, Dave was in the bedroom napping. I could count on at least two hours of peace and quiet. I'd just rented a steam cleaner and taken care of the worst of the carpet stains and was slowly making the house livable.

Popping in a CD, I began filling the dishwasher before tackling the stove and refrigerator—two cleaning chores I most detest.

"I have to throw up," Dave said, as he tottered on unsteady legs across the length of the house.

"There goes my window of opportunity," I thought. I turned to address my husband. "Dave, you don't need to tell me whenever you're feeling sick. Just throw up."

Instead of going back to the bathroom in our bedroom, or the half bath in the hall, Dave took me at my word and threw up. Right then and there. I turned away toward the sink, and he threw up. On me.

My first reaction was total and utter disgust. There I stood, dripping in chocolate vomit. I wanted to yell at him for taking me so literally but, of course, how would that help? I knew he hadn't done it on purpose.

Dave had perfect luck, or aim, since he didn't have a single drop on himself. After reaching for a cloth to wipe his face and making sure he was able to walk back to bed, I sent him on his way.

Now I had a dilemma. The chocolate-reeking vomit soaked through my shirt, making my skin clammy while I debated the best way to clean the mess.

Since I was in the kitchen with the easily-cleaned vinyl floor, I did what any woman would do in the same situation. I stripped, throwing my soiled clothes into the sink, and reached under the cabinet for the cleaning supplies. On all fours, armed with the pine-smelling liquid guaranteed to "disinfect as it cleaned," I couldn't help remembering a specific "Seinfeld" episode. If you haven't seen it, watch for the episode where Jerry questions good naked and bad naked. Trust me, this was the latter.

After cleaning the floor, I started toward the laundry room. There, I could not only wash the soiled clothes, but change into something freshly-washed from the laundry basket.

My house had a modern layout with all the rooms open and leading into one another. Normally, this would be fine. Today, however, it spelled disaster. To get from the kitchen to the laundry room, while carrying my smelly, wet garments, required that I pass the front door.

At the time, I lived in a lovely, single-family home in a suburban neighborhood. One of the nicest aspects of this subdivision was the security it afforded. It was such a safe place to live, I rarely locked my door.

Back then, Dave and I took advantage of his being ambulatory and still able to enjoy outings, so I took him out quite a bit. Because I got many deliveries and only locked the doors at night, the delivery people knew to ring the doorbell and, if no one answered, set the package inside the house.

My youngest son, Justin, whose nature is tenaciously curious, had dismantled the doorbell to see how it worked. He didn't put it back together perfectly and, as a result, the chime sounded only one short note—faintly. Preoccupied as I was to not drip chocolate on the newly cleaned carpet, I hadn't heard that one sickly chime. Just as I passed in front of the door, it flew open, and there stood the FedEx man.

That poor man. I'm sure as a delivery person in residential areas he sees a lot. I'm also sure he was nowhere near prepared for the sight of me naked, scurrying to the laundry room, reeking apparel clutched to my bare bosom. He quickly averted his eyes from my less-than-supermodel form, dropped the package, and ran. Funny thing, I never saw that particular delivery guy again.

What could I do? I continued my way to the laundry room, started a load of clothes with extra bleach, pulled on a covering, and made my way to the shower. Just another day with Huntington's Disease.

Eventually, I saw the humor in my story and shared it at an HD speaking engagement in Memphis. This city happens to be not only home to Graceland, Elvis Presley's home, but also to the FedEx corporate headquarters. Much of the audience either worked for FedEx or had a relative working there. Needless to say, they all got a good laugh.

The following month, Karen and Pam, two sisters from our support group who both work for FedEx, shared that they had written a letter to FedEx president, Fred Smith, requesting a donation for the cure. Of course I had to share my FedEx story and, again, everyone, including Dave, got a laugh.

A few months later, Pam announced that FedEx had made a generous donation to help find the cure for Huntington's Disease. A donation of $6,000 was presented to the Huntington's Disease Society of America. Karen and Pam like to think their well-worded plea was the reason for Fred Smith's generosity. I think that I possibly played a role in that donation. I've secretly decided that Fred Smith, or whichever vice president is in charge of corporate giving, must either be supremely compassionate or a breast man. Hey, whatever it takes! We have to do everything we can to find a cure. Even that. Thank you very much, FedEx!

"Shear" Survival

Expect a miracle!

—ANONYMOUS

Before either of my two younger sisters married, they shared a small house close to a small rural farm area in Houston, Texas. Diane preferred housework while Patricia agreed to take over the outdoor chores. At the time, Patricia worked and attended nursing school and usually arrived home when it was already too dark to mow the lawn. Weekends were no better and, eventually, the grass grew out of control.

"Patricia, look at the yard," complained Diane. "The grass is up to my waist. When are you going to cut it?"

"It's not that bad," Patricia exclaimed.

They walked into the backyard and, while the grass failed the waist-high test, it did touch their knees.

Patricia, determined to raze the burgeoning grass before it grew unmanageable, took a day off and got started early in the morning.

It didn't take long to figure out that the lawn mower couldn't quite cut it. The long grass twisted into the mower blades with each push. Hot and frustrated, Patricia considered her dilemma: how to hack down the tropical rain forest of a yard.

She didn't have a sickle, weed whacker, or anything even resembling a real garden tool. At her wits' end, Patricia called Diane at her office. "Diane, I can't do this anymore."

"Do what?"

"Cut the grass. It's too long and my hands hurt."

Confused, Diane asked, "What do you mean your hands hurt? How can they hurt just from using the lawn mower?"

Patricia, on the verge of tears, looked at her hands as she answered. "No. The grass is too high and thick. The blades won't move anymore."

"Then what are you using?"

In a small, tear-filled voice, Patricia answered. "Scissors."

No, she couldn't have heard right. "Scissors?"

Patricia had been using the sewing scissors to cut the grass. It wasn't long before blisters had formed as the scissor grips cut deeper into her flesh.

Diane, upon hearing the explanation, burst out laughing. "I'm sorry, Patricia, but I've never heard of anyone cutting grass with a pair of scissors."

In her air-conditioned office, Diane laughed. Patricia, at home and drenched in sweat, cried.

"I'm going to have to stop," admitted Patricia in defeat. "It's going to take a miracle to cut this grass."

Patricia spent the rest of the afternoon nursing her hands and staying cool. Diane continued working and neither of them thought much about the grass.

Later, as Diane pulled into the driveway of their small house, she was still chuckling about cutting grass with a small pair of scissors. "Only Patricia," she laughed as she headed to the backyard.

Rounding the corner of the house, Diane stopped short. "Patricia! Come out here," yelled Diane. "You're not going to believe this."

Running outside, Patricia stared first at Diane, then at the large animal in the backyard.

"Diane! Where did you get it?"

"I didn't get it. I got home and it was just here—eating the grass."

The girls gleefully laughed at their "miracle"—a cow eating the grass that had been too high to mow. Somehow, the hungry cow had wandered through the broken fence and into their yard from a neighboring farm. Everyone was happy. The cow, Diane, and especially Patricia, who had needed and received—a miracle.

Sometimes life with Huntington's Disease is exactly like cutting grass with a pair of scissors—the only way to survive is with a miracle.

Huntington's miracles come in all different shapes and sizes. Friends, family members, seeing humor in otherwise sad situations, and the right medication are just a few miracles that come our way when we need them the most. We all want a cure for Huntington's Disease but, until that day, look for the miracles.

Compassion

The impersonal hand of the government
can never replace the helping
hand of a neighbor.

—Hubert H. Humphrey

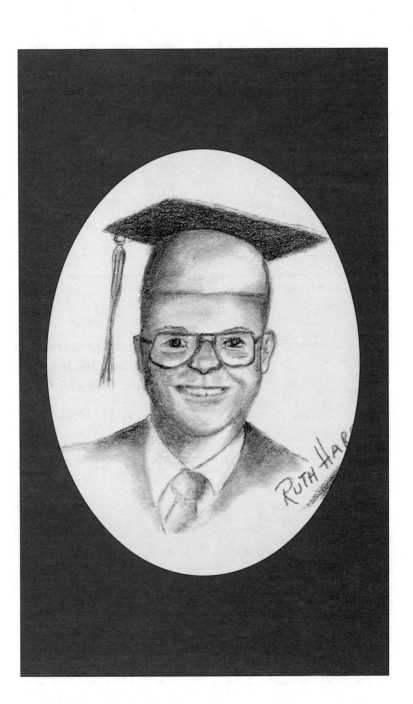

Always a Soldier

Resolve to be tender with the young, compassionate with the aged, sympathetic with the striving, and tolerant with the weak and wrong. Sometime in life you will have been all of these.

—BOB GODDARD

"When I grow up, I want to be in the army like Daddy," said Chucky LaFrance.

Mary smiled at the thought of her little man, all grown up and in uniform just like his father, Clarence LaFrance II. Clarence LaFrance III had a big name to live up to, but for now, he was just "Chucky."

"We'll see, baby," replied his mother. "You never know how life will turn out. But we need to be grateful for all we have, and use it well."

Perhaps Chucky's sweet disposition came from the proximity of his February 12, 1970 birthday to Valentine's Day. Chucky died February 11, 2001, still a sweetheart and still a soldier.

I talked to Mary today and cried. I wept for Clarence LaFrance III, and I wept for his mother, Mary.

I first met Mary Rush and her hospice nurse, Robin, at the 2000 Huntington's Disease Society of America convention in Orlando, Florida. They were like fertile soil, these ladies, thirstily soaking in as much information as possible, to give the best care to their Chucky.

One morning, as I exited my hotel room, I bumped into Mary. Chatting and walking to the elevator, it didn't take long to find out that Mary lived in New Orleans, as had my father and generations of his family. In fact, Mary knew of my grandmother and other family members of mine. Yes, it was a small world after all.

"I hear you travel around the country speaking about Huntington's Disease," said Mary. "I wish you could come to New Orleans. We don't have a support group or anything, but I want people to learn about Huntington's."

Mary went on to explain how, after over twenty years of dealing with Juvenile Huntington's, she had just learned of the Huntington's Disease Society of America. Once she heard there actually was a convention, her church had helped Mary and Robin attend their first gathering of Huntington's families. I could not believe she had dealt with Huntington's Disease all alone for such a long time. I knew I had to go to New Orleans, no matter what.

"I can do that," I assured her. "I have a convention in New Orleans this summer. I didn't plan on going, but I'll go, and I can visit you, too."

Whoever plans conventions in New Orleans in July has no compassion for those not enamored of hot, muggy weather. *I understand now why my father moved from this place,* I thought as I stood on the curb, waiting for my ride. "Lord, let them have air conditioning," I prayed as their car pulled up.

Mary and Chucky's step-father, Jimmy Rush, embody old-time, southern hospitality. Their generosity and openness made my experience in New Orleans enjoyable and special. While they couldn't take away the heat, they did everything else possible to ensure my comfort, even acting as my taxi drivers to and from meetings.

From our prior conversations, I knew enough about Chucky to understand he was in the final stages of Huntington's Disease. Knowing and seeing are completely different, so I took a deep breath as I prepared to meet Chucky. Upon entering their small home, I saw a large hospital bed that dominated the reassuringly cool room.

Despite his obvious weight loss and physical infirmities, Chucky flashed a brilliant smile and peered at me through slitted eyes. Mary stood next to me, every inch the proud mother. I held Chucky's hand, commenting on his soft skin and handsome face.

After a quick trip to the neighborhood fish market, Mary, Jimmy, and I settled around the table, peeling and eating succulent, spicy shrimp. We enjoyed the food while Mary shared Chucky's story.

Mary, the mother of two young children from a previous marriage, was thrilled when her second marriage resulted in a son. Named for his father, Mary knew that Chucky was destined to be special. "When he was only five years old I took him to see the doctor," remembers Mary. "Dr. Duncan explained to me about Huntington's Disease, and what was going to happen."

Sitting in the office that day, staring intently at his mother, Chucky, at times wiser than any child should be, simply said, "Okay. When God gives me a job to do, I have to finish it." He started with his neighborhood friends, telling them about God.

Chucky always lent a hand when needed. He had an inordinate amount of patience and compassion for others. His mother told me that Chucky took a lot of time helping with sick children. He encouraged others, regardless of their circumstances, to be better people and to love the Lord and each other.

Like so many people, Mary had never heard of Huntington's Disease before her little boy became symptomatic. "We never knew there was anything like this in the family. Looking back, I can think of others in the LaFrance family who probably had Huntington's Disease."

"I do remember," she continues, "that when Chucky's father came home from his first tour in Vietnam, he was not the man I remembered. He was abusive and angry. I told my mother I wanted a divorce."

Mary's mother convinced her to wait until Clarence came home for good. Post traumatic stress could easily have been the problem, she said, and Mary agreed to wait. Sadly, Clarence was killed in action and never returned.

"When I heard all the symptoms that could happen to my baby, I knew in my heart that Clarence had been suffering from Huntington's Disease and we never knew."

Despite knowing about his illness at such a young age, Chucky had a normal childhood. Children and adults alike enjoyed being around Chucky, especially his cousin, Trinette.

"My cousin, Chucky, and I are the same age, with only a month separating our birth dates," she says. "We were both born on the same days as successful men. My birthday is January 15, the same as Martin Luther King Jr., and Chucky's is on February 12, just like Abraham Lincoln."

Trinette and Chucky were together from nursery school through high school and were extremely close. Summers were spent at camp, and Trinette and her brother, Lammy, lived with Chucky's family to make it easier for them to attend. During high school, Chucky lived with their family.

Lammy remembers their times together. "He always liked to wrestle. I guess he thought he had the advantage, but I would get him when we boxed. In basketball, he thought he was Larry Byrd, and I thought I was Magic Johnson."

Chucky fell in love with a different beautiful girl every week. Looks were important, and he always loved the ones with long hair and pretty faces. Lammy remembers one girl in particular.

"I think Chucky was in love with this girl named LaQuita. She was my friend, and I always tried to hook them up."

According to Trinette, "Chucky was a good guy and never got into trouble. He enjoyed going out to the movies, watching television, eating out, and listening to music. We might have been cousins, but we were also best friends."

Trinette admired Chucky for knowing so much about his illness and wanted to make sure everyone else knew about it. "He never worried about the ramifications of the disease. He focused on the future and had dreams and hopes like anyone else."

Chucky dreamt of being a soldier in the army, which, of course, meant first graduating from high school. Despite increasing physical limitations, Chucky joined the ROTC and persevered. In fact, while I was in New Orleans, Chucky's ROTC instructor, Sergeant Major George Stimmons, came by the house to visit. He made glowing remarks about Chucky's character, attitude, and faith. Obviously, Chucky had made an impact on Major Stimmons. Here he was visiting ten years after graduation. Major Stimmons was one who paid tribute to this remarkable young man at his recent funeral service.

Chucky also dreamed of graduating from college. With the support of family and friends and a tenacious spirit, Chucky proudly graduated from the University of New Orleans.

Chucky's half siblings are both in the military. Abdul is in the Marines, stationed in Korea, and Sabrina is in the army in New Orleans. Sabrina's young children, Christopher and Kayla, would always drift back to Chucky's room and watch cartoons with him.

While Mary and her family might not have the support of a Huntington's Disease chapter or support group, many family, friends, and even teachers never wavered in their help and encouragement. Gail Matthews taught Chucky at L.B. Landry High School. "Chucky was an asset to me and all the students in my classroom. He was a pace setter. He always believed he could do anything that he put his mind to during his time on this earth."

Matthews remembers how Chucky encouraged his classmates to do their best. "'You had better finish your assignment,' he'd tell his friend. 'Boy, you better get an education and make something of yourself.'

"I often visited Clarence," his teacher continues, and talked to him about old times at school. I also told him I placed a picture of him in my classroom and told my present-day students his story. I told them of his strength and determination.

"I am proud of Clarence. I love him like a son. I am part of the family. I go to family activities, and Mary and I are good friends."

One of Chucky's other friends is Jerome Crosby, who remained a friend long after high school. "Chucky could do whatever he set his mind to. Having Huntington's was never an issue with him. Soon after he started at the University of New Orleans, he decided he wanted to learn to drive."

Chucky asked Jerome to teach him and Jerome willingly agreed. "We started out riding around the neighborhood. In no time at all, he was operating the gas and brakes on his own. He couldn't have been happier."

While many people can't relate to someone with a terminal illness, Jerome isn't one of them. Chucky's personality, faith, and innate goodness seemed to draw people like a magnet.

"I paid visits to Chucky as often as I could," says Jerome. "Whenever they needed money, I helped out to the best of my ability and as often as possible.

Jerome brought his wife, Lynelle, to visit too. "She first met Chucky at church where they had a program to honor him. Lynelle and I both continued to pray for Chucky and asked the Lord to give him strength."

The constant parade of people visiting Chucky while I was with them that week amazed and blessed me. Of course, the hospice nurse, Robin, came each day. You could tell there was a bond stronger than simply that of patient and nurse.

"When I first met Clarence, I was afraid I would not know how to care for him. He was completely different than my other patients in so many ways. It was hard at first because he could not communicate verbally."

Robin's fears were soon dispelled. "I could see he communicated through his eyes and bodily expressions. He also taught me more than I ever thought possible."

In fact, Robin honored Chucky, her favorite patient, in a time-proven manner when she named her baby daughter Clarice.

"Clarence's strong will and courage have inspired me greatly," insists Robin. "Seeing his mother care for him makes me hope I can care as much for my children as she does for her son. He touched my heart in so many ways, and I looked forward to seeing him every day."

A highlight of my trip to New Orleans came on Friday evening, when several of Chucky's relatives arrived at Mary's house to see Chucky and learn more about Huntington's. Mary was especially thrilled because, up until this point, the LaFrance side of the family seemed content to ignore the disease. We enjoyed the evening, and I told them all about Huntington's—sharing stories, singing songs, and answering questions.

Chucky's cousin, Jenetra, summed up everyone's feelings with her comments in a letter she later wrote to Chucky. "Every motivational thing I heard that evening has inspired me to look at your illness as a blessing and not with fear for our family. Now I know to live life to the fullest and not to complain so much."

When I talked to Mary today, she reminded me that the funeral took place only a week ago. It's amazing how empty a house can feel when someone who didn't even talk is no longer there. I heard such pain in Mary's voice, and I know her husband, Jimmy, feels it too. Jimmy loved Chucky and took care of him like his own son.

"I used to look forward to getting out of bed every morning and seeing that bright, beautiful smile," said Mary. "Seeing his smile let me know my day would be happy and bright.. I did all the talking, and he did all the listening—but with such a smile."

Everyone I spoke with that week in New Orleans, and everyone who later wrote a tribute to Chucky, mentioned an outstanding point—Chucky's faith. His faith carried him through difficult times, and he shared it with others every chance he got.

His Aunt Nancy wrote, "As Chucky's illness took a toll on his life, he never complained. He reminded me of a well-trained soldier, taking pride in the ROTC. Through good days and bad, that smile never faded."

Gentle and compassionate, Chucky cared that others would not be hurt by his illness. He made every effort to put people at ease and succeeded.

He graduated from high school and from college. Chucky's last dream was to be a soldier in the army. Some people would say it's a shame Chucky only achieved two of his three life goals, but that isn't true. As his Aunt Nancy said, "Truly, Clarence has always been, and will always be, a real soldier. A soldier in the army of God."

The Kama'aina and the Bread Stick Lady

The value of compassion cannot be over-emphasized. Anyone can criticize. It takes a true believer to be compassionate. No greater burden can be borne by an individual than to know no one cares or understands.

—BOB GODDARD

When we learned of Dave's diagnosis in 1994, I vowed he would have as full a life as possible and enjoy, for as long as possible, all that he had liked before we learned the news. He played on the church baseball team for awhile, but eventually moved to the stands to cheer them on to victory.

Even though we couldn't afford it, I gave in whenever Dave suggested a movie. I knew Dave would have a shorter time to enjoy life, and making it as full as possible became my goal. We've probably seen 95 percent of the movies released since Dave's diagnosis!

Dave's other love is food. Even now, pureed with little or no spice, Dave hungrily gobbles his meals as the hospice worker feeds him. Since the night we met, when Dave's gaze met mine at the Parents Without Partners meeting, his theme song has been, "I Only Have Eyes for You." Since his move to the nursing home, I'm not usually present at meal times because when I'm there, Dave stops all activity to stare. But I am still concerned that he gets enough calories.

Two breakfast burritos and a large Coke. That is how Dave started each morning in Hawaii once he stopped working. We'd walk or drive to the local McDonald's two blocks away, and Dave would always order the same thing. I'd suggest a different menu item or restaurant, but no, the world would end if Dave didn't get his two breakfast burritos and large Coke.

It didn't matter what was on my agenda each day, or even if I had the money, somehow I had to make sure Dave got his breakfast. We became a fixture, watching morning TV with the retired neighborhood cronies who chose McDonald's more for the coffee and companionship than the cuisine. Some days my schedule demanded visiting the drive-through window, but we always made sure we were there before the 10:30 breakfast cut-off time.

Clyde managed the restaurant, and we had a friendship based on my need to check out the huge yellow juice cooler filled with ice for various kid's soccer or basketball potlucks over the years. I'd sign the form promising him my first-born child if I didn't return the cooler. He'd hand me a jug of sweet, red punch syrup and a sleeve of small cups, emblazoned with the golden arches logo.

I knew Clyde as the kama'aina, or local, who managed the restaurant. He knew me as the mother of two Happy Meal-eating sons. He knew me as a team mom. Soon, he got to know me as the two-burritos-and-a-large-Coke lady. Each morning, whether at the drive-through or inside, Clyde watched as Dave and I did our breakfast routine.

One morning, the fateful day arrived: I didn't have enough money for Dave's breakfast. I offered to make him breakfast, but no, he had to have what he always had. I explained I didn't have any money, but that obsessiveness

111

that is often a part of Huntington's would not let it go. He wanted his standard fare, and he wanted it *now*.

Frustrated, tired, and feeling more than a little sorry for myself, I answered the phone on the third ring. "Where are you?" asked the vaguely-familiar voice.

"*Who* are you?" I countered.

"This is Clyde. From McDonald's. Where are you? Breakfast is almost over."

I explained we couldn't afford Dave's breakfast today because I didn't have enough money. I described Dave's tantrum at being denied, and Clyde quickly jumped in.

"If Dave wants breakfast at McDonald's every morning, he should have what he wants." This wonderful man, who knew me in only a superficial way, continued. "As long as Dave can eat, money will never be a problem. Come and get Dave's breakfast. I saved two burritos for him."

From that day until we moved two years later, Clyde was true to his word. Whether we ate inside or zipped through the drive through, we never paid. I don't know if Clyde took it out of his own pocket or if he used some creative bookkeeping to make Dave happy, but whatever he did, I will forever be grateful for his kindness.

I tearfully hugged Clyde on that last morning before we boarded the plane for Florida. I knew I'd never find anyone as kind as Clyde in Florida. Finances dictated that we had to move, so we left friends, family, and all that was familiar to begin a new life thousands of miles away.

About the time of the move, Dave's ability to swallow deteriorated to the point that no matter how much he asked, he wasn't getting a breakfast burrito. It simply wasn't safe. He still had a large Coke, but it was usually at the movie theater.

Once, after seeing a movie, we went to a restaurant that was new to me: Fazolli's. They bill themselves as Fazolli's: "real Italian, real fast," and while "real" Italian might be debatable, they are also "real" nice. We began to frequent Fazolli's even more after Dave entered the nursing home since it was convenient—right down the street. Dave could handle ravioli with an extra dollop of sauce once cut into manageable pieces. We made a glorious mess, but none of the staff ever made rude comments. Soon we were regulars with the counter help and the cheerful bread stick lady.

"You can't have any of this," she'd say laughing as she gently slapped Dave's hand away from the hot, yeasty roles. "You know you'll choke, and I can't deal with any dead people today." Her black humor made us both smile, and she'd bring him Coke refills and Italian ice, but no bread sticks.

One day, as we sat eating our meal, Dave coughed. If there was an Emmy or a Pulitzer for loud coughs, Dave would surely win. Patron's heads turned to look at the source of the thunderous noise. Whispered comments erupted and people pointed, but I ignored them and continued feeding Dave until, finally, their fascination ended.

Then, it happened. Dave coughed again, this time, louder than before and followed by a humongous sneeze! Now, if Dave's coughs rate an Emmy, his sneezes are a shoo-in for the Academy Award. When he sneezes, he does it with gusto, putting his entire body into it. And that day was no different. Unfortunately, that included his legs, and as he sneezed, I felt the table move. Before I could react, the table went flying,

People ducked to avoid the orbiting cups, plates, and splatters of marinara sauce. A cacophony of angry voices erupted: "Why is he out in public?" "Look at this mess. Don't they have places for these people?"

My heart broke for poor Dave as people angrily left their unfinished food and stomped out. The unkind comments were humiliating and undeserved. Just as I stood to tell these people what I thought of them, the bread stick lady began to speak.

"What's wrong with you people? So what if he made a mess. He's sick but he still deserves to live. Haven't you ever taken your children out? They make just as big a mess yet people call them cute. You ought to be ashamed of yourselves."

Her scathing comments, appropriate in my mind, had the desired effect. One by one, the chastised people quieted down, collected their belongings, and left. Without a word, the bread stick lady wheeled Dave to a fresh table, walked back to the counter, and brought us our lunch for the second time.

Those people at Fazolli's aren't the only ones who have laughed and made rude comments about Dave—and more are still to come. It's difficult to understand how people can be so insensitive. There are those who would argue that people have every right to expect a pleasant dining experience when they pay good money for a meal. Others might claim that their squeamish tummies don't allow for tolerance of less-than-perfect ambience. To these I ask: Why should the ill and their caregivers be closed behind doors and allowed into public only when those blessed with good health are not around? To these I offer a resounding, "Get real!"

Sometimes, when I most want to give up on the world, a Clyde or a bread stick lady will come along. In this tumultuous world called Huntington's, we've often had to count on the kindness of strangers to get us through one more day. I'm grateful that there are people who care, even in fast food restaurants.

A Heart as Big as Alaska

*Sympathy sees and says, "I'm sorry." Compassion sees
and says, "I'll help."*

—ANONYMOUS

I discovered a treasure named Marie one year before I
met her. Actually, I met her online, in a Christian Writers'
Group, before I finally saw her face-to-face. To some people, meeting online doesn't qualify as the real thing, but
though Marie lived in Colorado and I in Florida, our
friendship was strong even before we hugged each other at
the Denver airport.

In 1997 I decided to get more serious about my writing.
I had succeeded in selling a few magazine articles, but did-
n't feel I knew the craft of writing. Having recently moved
to a new state over 5,000 miles from home, I didn't have a
church or any type of support system; I felt disconnected.
Being the only caregiver for my terminally ill husband
made it difficult to get out of the house and meet people,
much less take a writing class.

The Christian Writers' Group, started as a ministry by
a dedicated writer and pastor's wife, is a forum for writers who communicate with each other via email. People
from all over the world join together to discuss writing
and publishing and support each other in prayer for both
personal and writing requests.

Unlike myself, Marie is what is called a "lurker." In Internet terms, this means she rarely posts messages but reads them all. In December of 1997, I asked for prayer; my brother, Merrill, was dying in Kansas. It was such a hard time. I really wanted to see him while he was living, and I wanted to take my sons to the funeral, too. But with little income, no medical insurance, and mounting bills, there was no money for airplane trips, no matter how important the cause.

Marie is not a wealthy woman, but her heart was touched. She gave me a gift that not only allowed me to see Merrill during his final days, but also to bring my sons back a week later for the funeral. While I was grateful to others who gave me modest gifts for the trip, I was overwhelmed when Marie sent her paycheck to me. She reasoned that she works because she likes to bless people, not because she needs the financial rewards of being employed.

Our friendship grew as we talked about our writing projects. *Faces of Huntington's* was my first book and was I ever excited. In her quiet, unobtrusive way, Marie began asking questions about Huntington's Disease. We exchanged information as our friendship grew.

As the book release date drew near, Marie's husband got a job transfer. Since they live in Grand Junction, Colorado, this meant a temporary separation while her husband, Ron, found an apartment in Colorado Springs. Ron moved about the time my books were ready for shipping from my publisher in Canada. The Huntington's Disease Society of America had its convention in Denver, and Marie graciously offered me space in their apartment. The plan was for my publisher to send a quantity of books there, to Colorado Springs. This represented a huge savings; I would not have to go through the expense and duress of lugging eighteen heavy boxes from Florida. All this, and we'd never met!

Marie drove all the way from Grand Junction, picked up the boxes, then met me at the airport where she promptly assumed the position of personal assistant for the next three days. She sold books, made change, answered questions, and was soon indispensable. All the while, she quietly soaked up information about Huntington's Disease and made several friends. I could never have made it without Marie, but each time I said thank you, she said, "No. Thank *you*!"

Recently, she told me that her life has never been the same since attending the HDSA convention. A few brief months before, she had never heard of HD. Now her life is changed. I knew it could be a life-changing experience for those with HD or in an HD family, but Marie is not affected personally by Huntington's Disease. She had never even met Dave.

An avid biker, Marie decided to raise funds for HD through biking. She and two friends, Charlotte Reicks and Evelyn Logan, made a trip that changed not only their own lives, but thousands more. These three women rode their bicycles over 3,000 miles.

In 1999, Marie and friends followed the old "Route 66" through California, Arizona, and New Mexico. They would continue through Colorado, Kansas, Missouri, Kentucky, West Virginia, Maryland, and into Arlington, Virginia, for the HDSA convention in Washington, D.C. By averaging approximately fifty miles a day, the trio reached their goal of 3,000 miles in two months.

Marie Nemec is a woman with a heart the size of Alaska. She told me she wanted to help by playing an active role in finding a cure for the thousands of people who daily live with this devastating disease. Help she did, not only on her first ride, but also the following year. In 2000, Marie rode her bike from California to Orlando, Florida. This year, she is planning a "border war" on HD. Her goal is to ride from the Canadian border to Tijuana, Mexico.

Marie created HD awareness and raised much-needed research funds. But, as much as I appreciate her willingness to ride those many miles for Huntington's Disease, there is something I treasure more. Besides sharing her friendship with me and biking for a cure, Marie does something even more important. Marie prays.

Sometimes the burdens of the world seem overwhelming. Marie aches for those who hurt and wants to solve the world's problems single-handedly. She probably wishes she had millions of dollars to help those in need. She doesn't have the money, and she can't solve all the world's problems, but she can and does pray. There is really nothing more significant that anyone can do for others than pray for them.

I'm so proud of Marie. And I'm honored to call her my friend. I'm thankful God led both Marie and I to the Christian Writers' Group. While I've learned much about writing and Christian publishing through the list, I've also learned that God does care and does provide friends for us in creative and timely ways. One reason I know this is because He provided for me through Marie.

Creative Solutions

The cynic says, "One man can't do anything." I say, "Only one man can do anything." One man interacting creatively with others can move the world.

—John W. Gardner

When I was nine years old, I started cooking for my siblings when our mom worked nights. She said working at the Menninger Foundation, a prestigious mental hospital in Topeka, Kansas, was more sane than staying home with eight children. Thanks, Mom.

Being a single parent with minimal child support, money was a constant problem at the over-stuffed white house on Munson Avenue. My mother always said, "We're not poor. We just don't have any money." It took me years to figure out what she meant.

Each day, I'd come home after school and take the single five-dollar bill my mother left in our hiding place. With the money, I'd go to the neighborhood IGA and buy groceries for that night's dinner. I'd also get soap, toilet paper, or any other needed items.

One day, though, there was no money in the normal place. "Mamma, where's the money?" I asked, calling her at work. It's a miracle she kept her job with all eight of us calling her two or three times a night each.

"Oh, darn! I forgot to leave it," she replied. I now know

she didn't forget; she simply had no money to leave. It was probably between paydays, and she needed the two or three dollars she had left to buy gasoline for the heap she drove.

"What are we supposed to eat?" I complained.

When Mom told me her plan, I wanted to die rather than carry it out. She repeated it twice more, then hung up, leaving me to wonder whether I really had to execute her plan or not.

Maybe it's because we had no pantry, but we kept our canned goods, at least most of them, in drawers. Where others had towels or other kitchen items, our drawers were a disorderly jumble of canned goods. I still think it's an odd place to keep green beans and beets.

I did as instructed. I opened the canned-goods drawer and pulled out vegetables, soup, and dog food, and placed them in a bag on the counter. When I finished choosing which items we could do without and which we needed, I carried the grocery-laden bag outside and placed it into the rusty, red wagon. I couldn't believe my mother wanted me to do this!

Her great plan for feeding us went like this. After choosing a reasonable number of canned goods, I was supposed to take the groceries to the neighborhood IGA. Once there, I needed to ask for the manager—beg him to trade the canned goods for whatever food we needed that night. Mom would never have asked a teenager to do it. After all, teenagers are always embarrassed about something and this really was embarrassing. Lucky for her, I was only ten.

I may have been just a kid, but even *I* knew the store manager wouldn't believe that this chubby kid, who looked like she had never missed a meal in her life, was really hungry enough to humiliate herself in front of people she actually knew. This could be a problem.

To ensure success, I asked—okay, demanded—my twin brothers join me in the great food trade. Michael and Merrill were only three or four at the time. With bare chests so the manager could see their ribs and stick-like arms, they walked into the store. Pulling two boys and the bag of groceries required more effort than I wanted to exert, so they walked until we got about a block from the store.

We finally arrived. I was out of breath and sweaty from pulling the wagon and my brothers.

"Look hungry," I urged my two unwilling partners. "Here comes the manager." Then to the manager, "We-don't-have-any-money-for-food-and-my-Mamma-wants-to-know-can-you-take-all-this-food-we-don't-need-and-give-us-stuff-for-dinner?" I asked breathlessly.

"What?" inquired the confused manager.

"We don't have any money for food, and my Mamma wants to know, can you take all this food we don't need and give us stuff for dinner?" I repeated my request, more slowly this time, while my brothers grinned maliciously at my embarrassment.

I honestly don't think he was taken in by my half-naked, emaciated brothers. I do think he was a nice man who understood my acute embarrassment.

A small group of shoppers listened intently as I explained my mother's plan. "Oh you poor thing," murmured on older woman. "I know your mamma works hard, but eight kids…."

Another customer chimed in and the manager handed me several dollar bills and some change in exchange for the canned goods. More kind-hearted ladies kept offering to buy us poor children food. Before I knew it, I had more than enough for not just one dinner, but several. Our booty included breakfast and lunch items, too. One kind soul even added ice cream.

My brothers insisted I drag them home, but the increased weight of the groceries made it impossible. Another wonderful soul loaded the wagon and groceries into her car and drove the triumphant warriors home. I don't remember what we ate that night, but I believe we had ice cream for dessert—and on a school night, too.

I recently saw my mother over the Christmas holidays and marveled at how young and healthy she looked. I don't think she could have survived single-parenting eight children without being flexible and willing to ask for help. Watching her tenacity and creative problem-solving has taught me to be a better parent and, not surprisingly, a better caregiver.

Having a husband with Huntington's Disease has been the most difficult thing I've ever experienced. Having no health insurance makes it even worse. There have been months on end when the money ran out far more quickly than the days of the month. And while I've never again tried to swap food at the local market, I have stood in line at food banks, solicited social service agencies to help pay utilities, and asked churches for help.

I've begged doctors to provide referrals for home health aides and asked friends and neighbors to take Dave to lunch, learn to use his feeding tube, and even asked strangers take him to the bathroom in public places.

I have not and will not let Dave go without the best care available just because resources aren't sufficient. I've learned there is always a solution to a problem and a way to fill a need. It might not be the most comfortable way of getting what is needed, but that doesn't matter. What matters is taking creative control over the situation and making sure those in our care with Huntington's Disease or any other devastating illness get all they need until there is a cure.

Pinches of Salt, Prisms of Light

The everyday kindness of the back roads more than makes up for the acts of greed in the headlines.

—CHARLES KURDT

Driving past my old house the other day I noticed the new landscaping. The sight of the first place I lived here in Florida brought back memories. I have been known to kill even silk plants and this spelled disaster for my suburban yard. To worsen things, by the time we had moved from Hawaii, Dave could no longer do yard work.

Continuing down the street, I looked at Diana's beautifully maintained plot and, smiling, remembered the day I'd first met her and became aware of her generosity.

"Hi Darlin'," Diana's honey-sweet voice had called as I walked back from the mailbox. "You mind if I plant some flowers round your tree?"

"Oh, that's fine," I answered. "Whatever you want. I just don't have any money for flowers."

How could I think about flowers when I was worrying about unpaid medical bills and car payments? We lived in a pleasant subdivision and, as much as I wanted to keep my yard looking attractive, I didn't have the tyme, tools, finances, or energy to make it a priority.

"Oh, don't bother about money," Diana assured me. "Your yard will look nicer when I'm done." I went about my routine and didn't think more about the yard.

Diana is exactly the sort of neighbor we all remember while growing up and is next to impossible to find in the suburbia of the new millennium. A lover of beauty, she delights in the outdoors. An offer of a few flowers soon grew to shrub-pulling, hedge-clipping, and trimming trees. Eventually, Diana started to cut my grass since I didn't own a lawn mower. She even talked my neighbor, Keith, into cutting my grass when he did his.

I made my way down the street, remembering Diana's kindness and my time at 569 Remington Oak Drive. Between Dave's illness and raising teenagers, it's a miracle I survived. Moving to Orlando from Hawaii, despite having no family or friends in the area, enabled us to live in a less-expensive area, but it also meant being without a support system.

In the beginning, I wondered how we could survive without that support system. Back in Hawaii, I was a respected member of the business community, active in my church, and had a thriving music ministry. The children had many friends, and Dave had others who cared about him. In Hawaii there was *aloha*.

Everyone has heard the word *aloha,* and most think it means hello or good-bye. Besides these meanings, the Hawaiian-English dictionary has over thirty meanings for the word. Some of these include charity, mercy, befriending, affection, love, hello, farewell, pity, endearment, friendship, sympathy, and hospitality. In other words, *aloha* is another word for being "salt and light."

The term salt and light comes from Matthew 5:13 in the Bible, but it's not only a biblical concept. Whether you call it the "Golden Rule," or simply being kind to each other, we are called to make a visible impact on the world around us.

I left *aloha* in Hawaii but soon discovered Central Florida has its own kind of *aloha*. For instance, moving used furniture 5,000 miles makes no financial sense. With very little money because of the staggering cost associated with illness and moving, we began frequenting garage sales and thrift stores. After many frustrations, a neighbor suggested we allow the Mustard Seed Furniture Bank to show us some *aloha*. In 1996 and 1997, over thirteen hundred families in Central Florida were provided with complete households of furniture. We were one of those fortunate families.

There are many other incidents of salt and light my family has received. Food, utility payments, and medical help were some of the larger displays. Equally appreciated were the kind words. There really are people filled with the *aloha* spirit no matter where you live.

A few years after arriving in Orlando, my friend, Eva Marie Everson, and I decided to write and compile a book of stories about being salt and light in the world. Writing stories from my own life helped me discover just how much salt and light I have received over the years. The book also gave me an opportunity to work with two special friends.

Erin Rettig and Soon Hee worked with me on my *Faces of Huntington's* musical CD, so I called them when it came time to create a musical CD for *Pinches of Salt, Prisms of Light*. Soon Hee is an incredible musician who captured the essence of the book in her song of the same title.

As a challenge, and with Soon Hee's kind permission, I've included the lyrics to her song. Rather than reflecting on relationships lost through Huntington's Disease, why not look at all who have been salt and light in your life?

S.H. Simmons once said, "Kindness is never wasted. If it has no effect on the recipient, at least it benefits the bestower." Online and face-to-face support groups, doctors, church members, social service workers, and countless others are salt and light. Hopefully salt and light bestowed on you has helped you cope with trying times. More than that, hopefully you've been, and continue to be, salt and light to others.

"Pinches of Salt, Prisms of Light"
by Soon Hee Newbold Rettig

In a world often heartless and cruel,
Where our children are grieving in school,
I look to the sky
And ask God "why oh why?"
How can we win the fight?
He softly whispers, "Pinches of Salt, Prisms of Light."

I don't know where to look or how to start
To see the world with the heart.
There seems to be no wrong or no right.
How can we win with only salt and only light?

Chorus

Pinches of Salt, Prisms of Light.
Spreading hope and faith through the night.
Pinches of Salt, Prisms of Light.
Only together can we win the fight.

As I look throughout the vast land,
I think I now understand.
Through the confusion, one part is clear;
We need to help each other with our every fear.

In trouble we soon forget our greed,
When a man stops to help someone in need.
A mother holds her child from a fall.
Maybe the world is not so bad after all.

Chorus

Bridge

Never give up, we're not alone,
We have an example, the way has been shown.
When the world seems dark by an endless night,
We are the Pinches of Salt, Prisms of Light.

Chorus

For more information about the *Pinches of Salt, Prisms of Light* CD, please visit http://www.writerspeaker.com or call 1-800-431-1579.

Faith

Faith is building on what you know is here,
so you can reach what you know is there.

—CULLEN HIGHTOWER

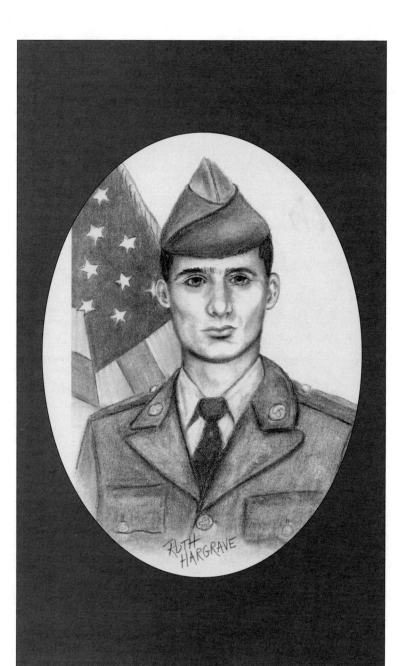

A Ministry of One

One filled with joy preaches without preaching.

—MOTHER TERESA

Loretta always knew her son, Marc, was destined for Christian ministry of some sort. Throughout his early teen years, even on days that she'd wanted to throw in the towel—or throttle him with it—she still knew God had called Marc for a special purpose. In his teens, Marc had loved attending church and youth retreats and, unlike many youngsters, had enjoyed reading his Bible. At sixteen, his only vacation souvenir was a picture of Jesus Christ, praying in Gethsemane.

Time has proven Loretta's ideas that Marc was somehow destined for ordination in the church, wrong. But Marc is still doing God's work.

When Loretta and Ron Church were married in 1974, she had been told that Ron's grandmother had Huntington's Disease. No one, though, had explained anything about it. Of course, in those days, little was known about it, and they themselves knew next to nothing about the disease that would ultimately change their lives forever.

When Marc and his fraternal twin, Scott, were born on July 15, 1975, Loretta was ecstatic. But over the years things began to change, and Loretta's happy life started a downward spiral that brought her pain and disillusionment,

133

even before there was an official title attached to Ron's worsening behavior.

"I thought I was living with a deeply depressed and angry man who chose not to do anything about it," she shares. "Now I know he was sick."

By the time the twins turned eighteen, she knew that their father had Huntington's Disease. Worse than that, she understood that each of her precious children had a fifty-fifty chance of having the gene themselves. Loretta asked them both if they wanted to be tested, but they each decided that they didn't want to know.

As Marc's symptoms increased, Loretta repeated this question. Again, he said no. Marc graduated from high school in 1993, then enlisted in the army. After three years of service, he received an honorable discharge after which he spent another year in the National Guard. Then Marc decided to follow his dream to be a pilot and, against his mother's wishes, joined the navy in 1998.

Loretta recalls her conversation with Marc when he decided to pursue his desire to fly. "When he made the decision to enter the navy, I told him he had a moral and ethical obligation to be tested so that he put no other sailors or citizens at risk because of his movements. Guns, bombs, and HD are not a good combination."

In hindsight, Loretta wishes she had stepped in and told the recruiter her concerns. Marc felt that this was his last opportunity to learn to fly, so off he went to the navy. Barely a month into training, he could no longer stand in formation and, facing the inevitable, Marc asked to be sent to a doctor. His sergeant sent him to a psychiatrist instead, believing Marc was just trying to escape serving his country. Thankfully, the psychiatrist who interviewed Marc saw immediately that he was sick and ordered tests that led to a correct diagnosis and an honorable medical discharge. A new chapter of his life and the lives of his family had begun.

Marc is blessed with a second caregiver in addition to Loretta—his step-father, David Bialas. A fire fighter who loves and cares for Marc alongside Loretta, David hurts, as any father would, to see his son suffer. David's teenage daughter, Amber, who cares deeply for her brother, is also having to watch as Marc's health slowly declines.

For Marc, the worst part of Huntington's is not the chorea or the inability to take care of his needs. It is the loneliness.

"Marc really misses going out with his friends for a couple of beers or a cup of strong coffee," says Loretta. "Instead, his day consists of watching television or listening to the radio. Mostly he stares into space in the dark. I often wonder what he is thinking about."

Marc's loneliness is something echoed by thousands of Huntington's sufferers around the world. In far too many cases, friends stop calling or coming over; their lives move on and there's no time to think about people like Marc who simply want a visit now and then. Loretta and David work hard to make Marc's life as full as possible, but it's difficult. It takes three qualities to make a difference; understanding, time, and love.

Those three qualities are what trained volunteers, known as Stephen ministers, have to offer. Marc was on a waiting list for quite a while before a volunteer named John, from Christ United Methodist Church, became a part of his life. Now they don't know what they would do without John, who Marc considers his best friend.

John, and other members of the Stephen ministry, prayed for a computer to help the family communicate with other Huntington's Disease families around the world. Through God's grace, a computer genius from the University of Texas built a computer for them. The computer and John provide Marc priceless comfort in the increasing loneliness of the disease.

Edwin Percy Whipple said, "Whenever you find humor, you find pathos close by his side," and this is true in this family. Certainly they have had their share of grief, but they also laugh.

When asked what sort of things provide them with this laughter, everyone agrees that since "pHD" is shorthand for "person with Huntington's Disease," they find it quite amusing that Marc got his "pHD" without attending college.

Marc's chorea has become a source of humor as well. Whenever Marc falls and his body jerks uncontrollably, he says, "I feel like a fish flapping out of water," and they all laugh hysterically.

Loretta remembers a not-so-funny time for her that had Marc laughing uncontrollably. "Marc loves to go to amusement parks and ride roller coasters. A year ago, we took Marc to the Fort Bend County Fair and he wanted to go on some of the rides. He could enjoy himself as long as we got him on and off the rides.

"I got him on one ride that spins around and goes up and down and makes you want to throw up," continues Loretta. "Just as I got Marc on the ride, the operator closed the door and I got stuck going on the ride with Marc. He thought it was so funny, and I was cursing my brains out yelling, 'I'm going to kill you when I get you home!'

"I felt awful telling my terminally ill son I would kill him, especially when I saw all the children listening to me while Marc was laughing. Unfortunately, I continued to cuss at him as the ride went faster and faster. It was a terrible ride, but it made Marc laugh."

Ultimately, the thing that gives Marc and his family the strength to get through one more day is their faith. Mother Teresa said, "I see God in every human being." That is exactly how Loretta feels.

"I see the face of God in Marc," says Loretta. "As I feed, bathe, and take care of him who is one of God's special children, I serve God."

Marc serves God by simply being Marc. He has come through the stages of grief and now accepts that he has Huntington's Disease and a cure might come too late for him. But he also knows that his life is far from over, and he still has a job to do.

With simple, childlike faith, Marc knows that having this particular terminal illness can be used to bring others to God. Marc is very serious about his love for the Lord, and he feels compelled to share it with everyone. He has given talks to several church youth groups and most recently, gave his testimony to a group of forty people at Calvary Baptist Church in Rosenberg, Texas.

Marc is very clear that his purpose in life is to bring glory and honor to God. He knows, without a doubt, others are seeing the face of Christ through this disease. Recently, Marc received a telephone call from the Fort Bend County Juvenile Probation Office, asking him if he would speak to the youth in their area. At the time of this writing, he was excited about talking to them and also about volunteering their home for youth community service.

Though her son's life has taken a different path than anyone could have anticipated, Loretta is as proud as any parent. "My favorite thing is to watch Marc with the neighborhood children, all five and under. They gather around him, and he takes them for rides on his wheelchair. They unabashedly give him kisses and hugs and their childish drawings. Their artwork adorns the walls of his room.

"Marc is sad that he will never have children of his own, but God has made sure that he does have children in his life," says Loretta. "He has often said that if one child, just one child, makes a choice to change his or her life, what a gift the world will be given."

People beyond Marc's family and neighbors also know what a special young man he is. At the HDSA 2000 convention in Orlando, Florida, Marc was given an award. The plaque says, "HDSA honors Mark Church, HDSA Person of the Year, for his example to others living with Huntington's Disease. June 10, 2000."

In a touching reversal from the normal-caregiver patient roles, Marc gave comfort to the caregivers at the last support-group meeting. Feeling tired and lonely, those caring for their loved ones with Huntington's Disease received a mini sermon.

"God challenges us to be more like Him," explained Marc. "If we become too comfortable in our own skin, then we cannot be open to change and acceptance." As usual, Marc was able to put things into proper perspective.

This remarkable young man is comfortable when talking about his mortality. To Marc, what ultimately matters is not how long you live, but what you do with your time on this earth. He also knows that God loves him and forgave him his sins.

I think Marc is hand-picking just who will spend eternity with him in heaven. He's hand-delivering invitations to them, one person at a time. Marc truly is in a godly ministry. Every day of his life.

The Treasure Box

You don't get to choose how you're going to die. Or when.
You can only decide how you're going to live. Now.

—JOAN BAER

Because my brother Merrill's song helped me find the theme of this book, I thought you might like to "meet" him and know what a wonderful brother I was blessed to have for thirty-six years.

Merrill died in January, 1998. A pastor, passionate about his ministry, he was only thirty-six. Far too young, most would say.

He was buried on January 12, the birthday he shared with Michael, his twin brother. At his funeral—a celebration, really—my oldest brother, Kevin, spoke of a dream he'd had a few days before Merrill entered the hospital for the last time. In his dream, he saw a box in heaven, engraved with Merrill's name and filled to the brim with gold coins. And on these coins were engraved the names of people he had led to the Lord, deeds he had done in the name of Jesus, people he had helped, and songs he had written.

As Kevin stepped closer and peered inside, he saw that the box was not just filled, it was filled to the point that not one more coin could be placed inside. Kevin awoke, knowing with certainty that Merrill, who had been ill off and on for four years, would be going home soon. You see, his treasure box was full, and God wanted him home. At thirty-six years of age, he had done all God required of him.

Merrill did more for God in the twenty or so years he lived for Jesus than most of us do in our entire lives. At the funeral, people stood and rejoiced at what he had meant to them. Telegrams from around the world spoke of his goodness, and over a thousand people crowded into the sanctuary of the borrowed church to honor this man. His own church, started five years previously, was too small. Churches throughout the city hosted meals for the family and congregation.

Tears were shed freely as we all realized we would never again hear his laughter, his music, or one of his messages. But tears of joy flowed just as freely as the stream of people who were saved because of his ministry came forward to tell their stories.

It was Benjamin Franklin who said, "Work as if you were to live one hundred years; pray as if you were to die tomorrow." That is exactly the way Merrill lived his life. He prayed, and he lived, as if he were to die tomorrow.

The "Glad Game"

Every cloud has a silver lining, but it is sometimes difficult to get it to the mint.

—DON MARQUIS

Dave has a devastating, degenerative disease for which there is no cure. The disease is slowly killing his brain cells, affecting his cognitive, emotional, and physical skills. He can do nothing for himself.

Cecilia lives in Namibia. Her husband, Steve, has Huntington's Disease, the same as Dave. When she first contacted me, I felt helpless reading her frantic email. While I didn't know anything about her faith, I did know that God had brought her into my life, through the Internet, from the other side of the world.

So I responded with a comforting message, letting her know that I understood. All the while I wondered how God would intervene.

Later that day, my friend, Linda, mentioned her son's mission trip to Namibia. Linda made arrangements through Sylvia, the pastor's wife in Namibia, to have someone visit Cecilia. I was comforted knowing that Cecilia, who desperately needed a friend, would soon have a visitor. I marveled at how quickly the Lord had responded to my heartfelt prayers.

Cecilia rejoiced at the news of the upcoming visit and

the care package I would send. Her hope and strength were renewed. She no longer felt as isolated. She knew I cared, and, now, she knew God cared, too.

Over the years, I've grown to admire Cecilia for her tenacity and her wonderful sense of humor. Just when it looked like she'd break from the pressure of caregiving, I'd receive a cyber card from her that usually had me in stitches. I knew Cecilia would survive.

Recently, my Namibian friend wrote to tell me Steve had passed away and is now in a far better place. God always provides, and while I've never met Cecilia in person and couldn't give her a hug during this time, I'm glad she has her special friend, Merryl, in Namibia.

As Merryl wrote in an email to Cecilia after hearing of Steve's passing, she thought of the "glad game" from the movie Pollyanna. In case you've never seen it, or you're a bit rusty on the plot, I'll fill in some details.

This 1960 Disney movie stars Hayley Mills as the little orphan girl, Pollyanna Whittier, who is sent back to the United States to live with her Aunt Polly after her parents' death. In the movie, Pollyanna tells the town preacher, Reverend Ford, how her father, a missionary preacher, taught from what he called the "glad texts" of the Bible. Pollyanna's father counted over 800 verses in the Bible where God tells us to rejoice or be glad or be happy. He decided that if God told us over 800 times that he wants us to rejoice, then He must be serious about being joyful.

Pollyanna also believed in playing the "glad game." Her father invented the game after Pollyanna had received a pair of crutches in a supply package. She had asked for a doll and cried when it didn't arrive. But her father told her they needed to look for something to be glad about. They both decided they were glad that they didn't need the crutches.

Now that you're familiar with the "glad game," here's Merryl's version.

Dear Cecilia,

I'm glad I had the opportunity to know Steve—the quiet, dry sense of humor and the person who was always welcoming, warm, and willing to share. Whether it was a task to be done, a cub outing, an opinion, his knowledge, a party, a beer, a quiet evening chatting, or a bottle of wine, he shared.

I'm glad that over the years, Steve was there for our meetings and various cub functions, always quietly taking responsibility for the money or tickets, but always efficient and present. That is how I best remember him.

I'm glad that in the early days after his illness was diagnosed, he was always invited to join in all activities and that it was his decision which to accept. I always felt special when he came here, and I am glad he felt comfortable enough to venture out of his safe home environment to visit us.

I'm glad that he was allowed the privilege of being nursed in a home environment, with people around who cared.

I'm glad for the fact that Christmas was so recent and that Steve could join in the traditional get-together of friends over sherry and mince pies, even if only for a short time. I'm glad that everyone there knew enough of Steve not to gawk awkwardly, but to welcome his presence. And I'm glad that he could enjoy that Christmas turkey, which obviously gave him so much pleasure.

I'm glad that he was spared a long stay in the hospital, linked to tubes and machines in order to stay alive for another lonely day without visitors, or worse, lying in a coma.

I'm glad that when the door finally opened for him, it was quick and easy and he was at home in his own room and bed where he felt most secure. I'm glad it was dignified and private.

And most of all, I'm glad that the time of waiting is over, that his suffering and private anger are finally at an end, and he is in a place of peace and love at last.

I'm glad that you have love and support to help you with a loss that we all feel and share. I know there will always be a special corner of your heart with Steve's name on it, where you will carry him forever.

There are many of you who have had to play the "glad game" when someone you love is no longer with you. I hope that one day, when there is a cure, you will remember to play this game for the other times in your life when there are disappointments. It really does make life more joyful.

Sweetness

The quality of a man's life is in direct proportion to his commitment to excellence, regardless of his chosen field of endeavor.

—VINCE LOMBARDI

Years ago, I lived in Mt. Prospect, a northwestern suburb of Chicago. During that time, I was pregnant with my first child, Nicholas, and had an obstetrician in Schaumburg, Illinois.

For several months, the sweetest man would accompany his pregnant wife to that same clinic, and he and I became good waiting-room buddies. It turns out this lovely man was Walter Payton, the football player and running back for the Chicago Bears.

Walter was the softest-spoken, sweetest guy, and it's easy for me to see how he earned the nickname "Sweetness." His wife and I eventually had our babies, and I never saw Walter again in Chicago.

Fast forward several years to Hawaii, where I moved less than a year after having my son. I attended a business function held at the grand opening of a restaurant called Studebaker's. No sooner had I walked in than I heard someone asking, "How's that boy of yours?"

I had no clue who was asking about my son, but it was Walter Payton, now part owner of Studebaker's. We chatted about our kids and our lives and he gave me his autograph.

I still can't believe he remembered me with all the people he must have met over the years. I'll never forget what an absolutely wonderful man he was, with a tremendous faith in God.

Walter had become the National Football League's all-time leading rusher and led the Bears to win a Super Bowl championship.

Coincidentally, we had another connection as well. Walter died November 1, 2000 of *primary sclerosing cholangitis*—a rare liver disease that could only be cured by a transplant. He waited nine months and never got that transplant. My brother, Merrill, a pastor and a singer with a breath-taking voice, also had *primary sclerosing cholangitis.*

In January of 1998, at the age of 36, Merrill passed away. Merrill loved football, and he also loved Walter Payton. They both had such sweet spirits and were each major practical jokers.

I'm sure they are having a ball up there, singing, joking, and tormenting my dad, who died in September of 2000. You see, my dad was anything but a Bears fan. My dad loved football, too, but went for the Kansas City Chiefs all the way. The last time I saw my dad alive was at Merrill's funeral.

Walter Payton won respect for carrying the football, Merrill for being a pastor, and my dad for his years of service at the post office. All three were admired even more for the way they lived their daily lives.

NFL Commissioner Paul Tagliabue said, "Walter exemplified class, and all of us in sports should honor him by striving to perpetuate his standard of excellence. The tremendous grace and dignity he displayed in his final months reminded us again why 'Sweetness' was the perfect nickname for Walter Payton."

I think all of us should honor Walter whether we're in sports or not. He exemplified how we should all live, no matter what our jobs or our situation in life. I mourn the passing of these three men who earned my admiration by the way they lived.

I also mourn the passing of too many who have died from complications of Huntington's Disease. The courage and dignity these incredible people have displayed throughout their illness has been an encouragement to me, their families, and others whose lives have been touched by them. Just as I honor these three men in this story, I pay tribute to all who have lost their battle but are now in a better place.

The Bracelet Promise

Faith may be defined briefly as an illogical belief in the occurrence of the improbable.

—H. L. MENCKEN

Since I began writing four years ago, I have written many stories. Some have been about Huntington's Disease, while others have been about life experiences that have nothing to do with Huntington's or any illness at all.

Of all that I have written, though, the story people love the most is, "The Bracelet Promise." This story has been published in several magazines, web sites, and compilation books. Many people around the world first heard about Huntington's Disease because they read this story.

As I travel and speak around the country, I am often asked about the bracelet. It is truly one of my most prized possessions, not because of its beauty or value but because each time I see it, I remember the special times with Dave.

It's also the story that kicked off my writing career. Our first December in Florida, I sat down to write my annual Christmas letter. As I skimmed my friend's "brag letters," I grew more and more depressed. Why was my life so horrible? The letter I wanted to write went something like this:

> Aloha from Florida. We were forced to move from our island paradise because of a hideous disease called Huntington's. The high cost of living, coupled with a lack of appropriate nursing homes for the future, made

living in Hawaii an impossibility. In the process, we lost our home and have no family or friends here in this hot, humid hell-hole. My kids are angry and doing terribly in school. Dave continues to decline and I've never been so unhappy in my life!

Well, that obviously was not going to make anyone's holiday cheerful, so I quickly threw that letter away and started over. I thought about it for a few days but still couldn't decide what to write.

One day, a stranger commented on my bracelet. As I told her the story, I realized things weren't as terrible as my pity-party made them look. They were almost as bad, but that didn't mean they wouldn't get better. I still had the promises that the bracelet represented.

I went home and wrote my Christmas letter, which was actually this story. People emailed, wrote, and called after receiving the story, and they all said the same thing. Write more! That is how Faces of Huntington's began.

Because some of you have never read Faces of Huntington's, or you might give this book as a gift to someone who has never read the story, I'm including it next. At the end of the story I've included an addendum you might enjoy....

The glitter of green stones drew me to the solitary display case. Light bounced off the silver and glass. Amidst the jumble of holiday shoppers, I made my way to the corner area reserved for fine jewelry and gazed upon the bracelet, noticing its unique handiwork. The beaten silver, fashioned in such a way as to resemble diamond chips, was delightful. Seeing dozens of dark green emeralds, I knew this was a one-of-a-kind treasure.

As I stared in wonder at the intricate piece, I remembered a promise my husband had made. David had bought me a lovely gift four years earlier on our honey-moon. He had selected an emerald green, Austrian crys-tal and seed pearl bracelet in honor of my May birth-stone. As he fastened it on my wrist, he lovingly said, "I promise that soon I will buy you real emeralds. Just wait." Though I loved the honeymoon gift, deep down, I looked forward to David's promise.

Until that time, however, I still delighted in wearing the delicate creation. I wore it frequently, each time remembering the island boutique. Whenever David saw the bracelet, he remembered his promise and would reas-sure me that the time was coming soon when he would keep it.

It became our habit over the years to look in every jew-elry store window as if searching for the Holy Grail. We wandered in and out of countless shops, becoming dis-couraged when we realized that the cost of the promise was well beyond our means. I soon wavered in my belief that I would ever own what David desired to give me. David, however, never lost faith.

Now, we were in the mall during the last week before Christmas to buy gifts for our children. Finances were tight, so we agreed there would be no exchange of gifts between us. We had just completed one of the most stress-ful years possible. With David's diagnosis of Huntington's Disease, our lives had forever changed. This terminal, neurological disorder pitched us into a panic, not to men-tion near bankruptcy.

I looked up from the case into David's eyes and saw love shining even brighter than the stones. I could read his mind: nothing short of this bracelet would satisfy his honeymoon promise. I also knew there was no way we could possibly afford it. I tried to tell him, but the words died on my lips. He'd had so many disappointments that year, I didn't have the heart to tell him the answer was "no."

Thinking fast, I came up with a reason to decline what I knew was an offer I could not accept. I have large wrists and normally bracelets don't fit. As the store clerk reverently lifted the object out of the case, I knew it would be too small.

The silver and green made a colorful contrast against my brown skin, and I silently acknowledged how much I wanted this bracelet, all the while hoping it would not fit. As the clerk reached around my wrist and closed the intricate clasp, my heart both plummeted and leapt. It fit! It was perfect, yet I knew there was no way we could afford it. The unpaid bills, with the promise of more looming in the future, had placed a vise around our checkbook.

I glanced at my best friend and saw his shining smile burst forth. This man, who had never hurt anyone, was now the victim of one of the cruelest diseases known to man. His was a sentence with only one verdict—death. An untimely, slow, and cruel death. My eyes brimmed over with tears as I realized we would not live out our dream of growing old together. To David, this was not just one more bauble in an already overcrowded jewelry box. Rather, this was his love displayed on my arm for all the world to see. To David, a promise made was a promise kept. I sadly realized that he might not have many more months or years to keep his promise. Suddenly it became the most important covenant ever made. I had to juggle the bills to let him have the honor of keeping his promise.

"Do you like it?" he whispered. Hearing the hope in his voice, seeing the love in his eyes, was something I am sure few women have ever had the privilege of experiencing. It was clear that David cherished me. All he had ever wanted, from the day we met, was to please me.

"Yes, honey, I love it," I answered. "It's exactly what I want."

The clerk reached for my arm to remove the bracelet. I could not believe that this little object had worked its way into my heart so quickly. "How much is it?" I finally asked. Slowly the man turned over the little white tag. Two-hundred-fifty dollars it read. Surely it was a mistake! I had seen enough emeralds in our searching to know that price was only a fraction of its worth.

The man began to extol the virtues of the item, pointing out the hundred and eighty emeralds in a hand-made Brazilian setting. But even though 250 dollars was an incredible price, it might as well have been 2,500 dollars for all we could stretch our meager budget. Without thinking I asked, "Would you take 225 dollars, tax included?" I surprised myself at that question because shops in malls do not normally bargain. He looked at me in surprise and answered, "That will be fine."

Before he could change his mind, I whipped out my credit card, all the while watching as David beamed with pride. The man quickly handled the transaction, and we were on our way. Every few steps we would stop and look at the bracelet. Before we reached the car, David said, "When I get sicker and eventually die, you need to look at each emerald. Each one will remind you of something special we've done. A trip we took, a movie we saw, or a moment we shared. This will be your memory bracelet." I began to cry. David's concern was not his own failing health, but how I would handle life without him.

As we worked our way home in the bumper-to-bumper traffic in rush hour Honolulu, I wondered just how we could pay for the bracelet. Oddly enough, I never really panicked. I was just curious as to how it would all work out. We talked as we traveled and every so often looked at the miracle of the promise kept.

On the way into the house, I grabbed the mail and began to open it as we walked. Amidst the usual bills were two cards. I opened the first which was from a church where I had sung several times that year. It was a thank-you note for my music ministry along with a gift. I was speechless. I was looking at a check for 200 dollars! I reached for the second card and slit it open. Out fell two bills—a twenty and a five. The card was simply signed, "A friend in Christ."

I looked up at David and we both began to laugh. I remembered how I had felt the need to ask the clerk if he would take 225 dollars, tax included. Even as we were in the mall, the payment for David's promise was in the mailbox. God had already taken care of every detail, including the twenty-five dollars plus tax.

It is just a piece of jewelry, something I could have lived without. But the memories attached to our time together have helped make me the woman I am today. The exquisite joy and the unspeakable grief of this relationship have grown me in ways I could never have anticipated. The promise David spoke on our honeymoon had been fulfilled. It was only through God that we stopped at that shop on that day to find that specific bracelet. The pastor of a small church, coupled with an unknown friend, listened to God as they decided their holiday giving.

Before I was ever born, God made another promise. He promised me eternal salvation. He promised He would be with me every step of the way. All I had to do was ask. Just as God never stopped believing I would claim that first promise, David never stopped believing in his bracelet promise. When I wear my emeralds, I pull out memories that are tucked away in my heart. I also remember David's faith—and God's promises.

A few months after Faces of Huntington's was published, I asked a jeweler about my bracelet. I told him I didn't want an appraisal, but wondered how much he would want for something similar. He took out his jeweler's loupe and carefully examined the bracelet.

After telling me this was only an estimate, he suggested the bracelet would sell for 2,000 dollars! I laughingly told him he had made a mistake. No, he assured me, it would be close to that price.

As I walked away from the store, I realized what must have happened. The original prize was 250 dollars. I think someone accidentally left off the second zero and the sales clerk never noticed.

I hope no one got into trouble over that mistake, but this just makes it even more obvious that the bracelet promise was meant to be. Dave had faith he would find the perfect bracelet. Each time I look at his precious gift to me, I realize God is at work in this disease, and I have faith that we will find a cure. Isn't God good?

Love

———————————————

*If you judge people, you have
no time to love them.*

—MOTHER TERESA

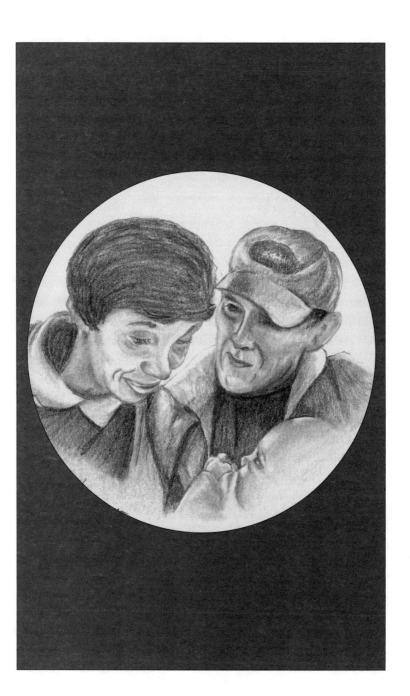

Anniversaries

Love at first sight is easy to understand. It's when two people have been looking at each other for years that it becomes a miracle.

—SAM LEVENSON

Mary Martinot gave birth to Rose out of wedlock. Mary's promiscuity resulted in many half siblings for Rose, but Rose had the good fortune to be adopted by a family who lived nearby—Gregory and Mae Cabral. Mary visited Rose a few times, then disappeared. They later discovered that Mary had spent the last fifteen years of her life in the state mental hospital. Ironically, at one time, Rose had lived less than two blocks from her mother and never knew it.

Rose Cabral had a happy childhood, and her adoptive parents created a very loving, supportive environment, even though both were old enough to be her grandparents. Raised as a Catholic, she attended a multi-racial Catholic school in the Roxbury section of Boston.

After graduation, Rose went to work as a secretary for a financial consultant in Boston, and later as a secretary in the labor and delivery ward where, ironically, she later gave birth to her children.

Ken Shears called Albuquerque, New Mexico home. As an only child, Ken remembers spending time in nursing homes where his mother worked. A product of the sixties,

Ken was a conscientious objector during Vietnam, but in lieu of serving his country in military service, Ken worked at a hospital in Oklahoma City, Oklahoma. Finally, following a trip to Europe, he stopped over in Boston, Massachusetts and decided to settle down there.

Then, twenty-seven years ago, Ken and Rose met on a sunny spring day. A few short months later on the Esplanade in Boston in front of the Hatch Shell, Ken proposed to Rose. "I wasn't even sure I loved her," confesses Ken. "I just knew she was the girl for me."

They were children of the times, "taboo breakers," as Ken calls it. He is white; she is black. Rose had been raised by adoptive black parents in Roxbury, but years later, while searching for answers, they discovered that her dad was indeed a "handsome black man from Jamaica," her mother, a white woman of Lithuanian descent from South Boston.

So, on June 15, 1973, they married. Mixed marriages were not the norm then, and this young couple bravely faced what seemed like the entire gawking city of Boston. Ken says, "We clung together like two people in our own small life raft on the high seas of hatred."

Despite the hate, or maybe because of it, their love grew and became their life preserver. Nine months later, the birth of their daughter, Helene, ruined Ken's first day with the telephone company. He didn't make it through the shift because he was Rose's "coach." A year and half later, their son, Matthew, was born, followed several years later by the birth of Jackie. Three more anniversaries to celebrate each year.

When Rose first started showing signs of Huntington's Disease, they were clueless. There were subtle changes in

Rose which, later, they knew had been the first signs. "She didn't become a different person or start acting in grossly different ways than she had before," explains Ken. "It was simply a matter of her behavior becoming inexplicably magnified. She began to feel things and express those feelings more forcefully. There was an increase in emotion, anger, and sentimentality. What had previously passed as minutia, small or unimportant details, now became hurdles that seemed to be rising daily."

With no knowledge of family background, Rose and Ken were spared the fear, frustration, and anger related to being at risk. "At first I thought she was going through the whopper of all mid-life changes. A long, agonizing [pre-gene discovery] series of tests eventually revealed the truth. When the day arrived, this ex-Catholic girl and her ex-atheist husband cried out to God in the neurologist's parking lot, our heads ringing with the words: 'Huntington's Disease, incurable, and genetic.'"

Last year, Ken and Rose celebrated their twenty-sixth wedding anniversary. He took some time off work and lunched with Rose. They passed a pizza parlor, and she said "pizza," so, pizza it was. It was followed by ice cream. As they enjoyed their pizza, Rose kept saying "I love pizza." Normally, she says only one word, sometimes two. To string three words together is a real achievement. In the midst of keeping her from burning herself on piping hot pizza, then keeping her from choking on the gooey stuff, Ken leaned in as she paused and clearly said, "I love you."

"It is easy to dream of an anniversary meal served at a fine restaurant on beautiful china with the best service. Nothing shall ever compare to being in the back seat of our Dodge, covered in pizza and ice cream, with my beautiful Rose. Being told by the only person who has ever really mattered to me, not counting my wonderful children, that I was loved makes life not just bearable or "worth living," but for me, it makes life outrageously magnificent."

Several months have passed since an anniversary Ken and Rose didn't celebrate. Over three years ago, Ken moved Rose into a nursing home where her needs could be best met. While the guilt still lingers that Rose is no longer at home, Ken persists as an active caregiver, even moving to the town where the nursing home is located.

"I relocated to be closer to her nursing home, only to discover that instead of visiting her everyday, as I had planned, I visit only slightly more often than I did when we were further apart. Still, it has been so ordered that I pass Rose every day going to and from work. When I gaze at her second story window, I see only reflected sky. Behind that reflection sits my beautiful wife in her Broda chair, or, perhaps she is lying in her bed, looking into the same sky that paints her window."

Where others see a person ravaged by disease, Ken sees only beauty. "In some wondrous way I've been blinded by Rose. She so saturates my life that time apart is still time with her. She is ever present, a flickering light always in the corner of my dimming eye."

Ken and Rose have, as do all couples, many anniversaries to celebrate. The anniversary of their marriage, of the births of each of their three children, and now of their grandchild. Even the anniversary of the date their last child was lost before being born is an important one.

"As hard a time as that was," says Ken, "it brought me to Jesus Christ. Rose later said that she was sure that was the baby with HD. She believed with all her heart that our kids are all free of the disease."

Some anniversaries are remembered but not celebrated. Probably the day of Rose's diagnosis is one such date, as is the date she moved into the nursing home. Without a doubt, that March in 1973 is the anniversary of a great love story between Rose and Ken....

"Rose is the only reason I know how to express love; she stands at the absolute center of my life. Though ill and but a shadow of her former self, her power to love is undiminished."

I'm sure that if Rose could speak, she would utter the same loving tribute to her Ken.

Expressions of Love
by Ken Shears

*A mother is not a person to lean on but a person to make
leaning unnecessary.*

—DOROTHY CANFIELD FISHER

After many years of overwhelming personal difficulty,
our daughters are now able to relate much better to their
mom. Maybe it's because Rose now relies on them fully
when we visit her or bring her home from the nursing home.

Jackie, our youngest daughter, constantly refers to her
mom as "sweet" and loves her very much. She laments not
having a mom with whom she can share her triumphs and
tragedies with on a normal basis. Still, Rose and I are so fortunate; as a result of the pain caused by Huntington's, Jackie
and her older sister are close in ways that transcend sister-
hood. They also correct erroneous memories I have of how
Rose did her housekeeping and myriad other details that
spring from youthful recollections of their mother before she
became ill. They're beginning to realize what they owe her.

We have, like all families, shed many a tear over our
losses. But we are also blessed by the wonderful memories
we made before Rose became ill.

There's an acronym used in the Christian teen community: "WWJD." It stands for, "What would Jesus do?" For
our children, it's WWMD or, "What would Mom do?" Our

kids constantly correct my memories about what their mom liked to eat and how to fix it. I'm a terrible cook and, boy, do they let me know when I fall short of the mark! They also correct myriad other details that spring from their youthful impressions of their mother before she became ill.

Our house is full of the crafts Rose created, offering unbroken links to her love. These are silent icons of her attention to detail we rarely noticed at the time, but which now stand as beacons of her love and care for all of us.

We are blessed to have reached the point where we can meaningfully return the love she so richly deserves. Even though Rose is now in a condition that some would call helpless, she is still the focal point of our family.

Last year, I was hospitalized because of cancer for a total of two months. I had two radical procedures performed during that time and, for awhile, things were "touch and go." Looking back, though, what I remember most vividly was the comfort of having my children, people from my church, and even hospital staff simply hold my hand.

But in a twist of fate, I was most comforted by my wonderful Rose, whom I'd had to place in a nursing home just a few months before. I'd visited her a few days prior to my last hospitalization, and, unsure she would understand what I was trying to tell her, I bluntly explained my situation. She quietly leaned forward and pressed her forehead against mine. Though Huntington's Disease has almost totally robbed her of speech, this expression of her love did more to erase my despair than any words she could have spoken.

We are continually learning to share our feelings, to show our love. I sincerely believe that, however difficult it may be, honestly and simply sharing your feelings for another's suffering is a precious gift that outlasts all the tears and fears.

Wooden Spoons

Love does not dominate; it cultivates.

—GOETHE

"Mom, you can open your present," Justin exclaimed, "but only if you promise not to use it on me." The festive Christmas package, proudly yet childishly wrapped, did little to conceal the shape of the present so carefully chosen by my four-year-old.

Justin's eyes shone with excitement as he waited for the moment when I would unveil his treasure.

"See, Mom, they're wooden spoons. You need 'em to cook, but you gotta promise you won't spank me with 'em."

I can still see the earnest expression as he offered me his gift—with strings attached. Though I continued, on occasion, to use wooden spoons to lovingly mete out his discipline, I never used those spoons. Now, almost fourteen years later, the spoons are broken or have been lost in moving.

In recent years, during family weddings and funerals or just because, I unwrap memories of my children that I keep tucked away within myself. Most of them are sentimental or funny, but some of them I wish had never happened.

Most of the unhappy memories happened after Dave, my sons' step-father, became symptomatic with Huntington's Disease. Even though they are not at risk for Huntington's, my boys are still affected. It's impossible to live in a family where a parent has HD and not be impacted.

My older son, Nicholas, does not like Florida. Angry at the move from his father and his island life and friends, he could have rebelled as many teenagers do. Instead, Nicholas reacted to the move and the unhappy times in our home with typical determination, and became a better student.

Naturally intelligent, Nicholas began to read the classics, as well as a huge variety of literature. He became an "A" student, where previously he had lagged in math. The biggest change, though, came in his senior year.

Because I benefitted from being an exchange student to Brazil while in high school, I wanted my children to do the same. Back when life was "normal" at home, I had talked to Nicholas about the program. He responded by claiming that he would never live in a stranger's house, eat food he didn't like, or learn a new language. His comfort level on Oahu would keep him in America.

Settling into Florida challenged everyone, and our collective stress, if measured on a richter scale, probably reached the upper limits. Eventually, Nicholas decided that living with a new family in a foreign country was preferable to staying in Florida and dealing with all the problems of Huntington's Disease. Ouch!

Not only did Nicholas study overseas, he went to a country he had never even considered before. I doubt he would have done that had he been happy, but he went to the Czech Republic and discovered an innate capacity for learning foreign languages we never knew existed. He now speaks fluent Czech, is quite good at German, and is interested in other Eastern and Central European languages.

As a result of his foreign study with the AFS program, Nicholas received a large scholarship to a prestigious private college. He has since traveled back to the Czech Republic and will be attending a semester of his junior year at a Czech university. Ultimately, his plans include using his Czech and political science interests as a jumping-off point for a career. None of this would have happened had we not had Huntington's Disease in our family.

My younger son handled his stress and anger differently. His grades plummeted, he dabbled with drugs and tobacco, and chose the worse class of friends available. His rebellion, on top of Dave's illness, at times became more than I thought I could handle.

Justin is now a senior in high school but doesn't live with me because of choices he made. Yes, in a perfect world, he would have known I loved him and not taken so much that happened with Dave personally. In other words, he should have hated the disease, not the person. But he was only a little boy when it all started, and then an adolescent who was unwilling or unable to open up and talk about his feelings.

Eventually, he chose to spend his final year in high school back in Hawaii living with his father. While I feel cheated in some ways to be missing his senior year after all we went through, I also know Justin had to deal with the issues surrounding HD in his own way.

The other day while talking to Justin on the phone, he said he was proud of me. Surprised, I asked him why.

"I'm proud of you now, Mom. You are writing and speaking to help people that you wish you had never heard of. I know how Huntington's has hurt you, but you are still helping people." With surprising emotion, Justin continued. "I'm proud that you survived the Huntington's years with Dave and two hormonal, angry teenagers in the house. I don't know how you did it."

This is very insightful for a seventeen year old—insight gained through a lot of hurt and, now, through seeing things from a distance. Do I wish Dave had never gotten sick and that my family had stayed intact? Of course I do. But I can't control most of what goes on around me. I think ultimately both of my sons will be better men because of all they have gone through, but it was not easy or pleasant for any of us.

I used to play the "what if" game, trying to figure out what I could have done to help my children better understand what was happening in our home. What if Dave had moved to the nursing home sooner? What if I had gone on welfare back home and not moved? What if I had devoted every minute to my kids and Dave and none to myself and others? What if, what if, what if….

Of course, I finally realized that "what ifs" are pointless and usually make for crippling guilt feelings.

I still appreciate Justin's Christmas gift from so many years ago. Even though he gave me those spoons with strings attached, I never used Justin's wooden spoons to spank either of my children, but I did use them for cooking meals and treats for my family.

My sons and Dave love my cooking. They sometimes ask why I can use the same ingredients as other people but still my food tastes better. I tell them it's because I add love to my food.

There are many things I've done wrong in dealing with situations in my family. One thing I have tried and usually succeeded at, is showing that with my love, there really are no strings attached.

I'll Love You Forever

The great gift of family is to be intimately acquainted with people you might never even introduce yourself to, had life not done it for you.

—KENDALL HAILEY

One evening, I was playing Monopoly with a family friend and my sons, fourteen-year-old Justin and sixteen-year-old Nicholas. The game was going smoothly until Justin, in a characteristic, major capitalistic move, wanted to buy several properties from his brother. This coup, if he could coerce his brother into selling, would give him a monopoly: one entire city block.

This was bad news for the other three players in the game. I was perilously close to bankruptcy. So Justin offered his brother an obscene amount of money, to no avail. When that didn't work, he switched to incentives, including, "You'll never have to pay me rent if you land on these." Nicholas, child of my heart during that hard-fought Monopoly game, persisted in saying, "No."

Finally, Justin looked at his brother, often the source of such conflict and jealously in his life, and smiled. "Please let me buy them from you, Nicholas. If you do, I'll love you forever."

Nicholas' face melted, and we all broke into laughter. Their completed transaction soon forced me into bankruptcy,

170

and the game eventually ended with Justin the undisputed real estate mogul, despite not charging his brother rent.

Sometimes, life is challenging at best, and a nightmare at worst. But whenever I see my kids together, so handsome and strong and so close to being on their own, I hear Justin saying, "But I'll love you forever!" I know it's true, and those words get me through one more rough day.

My Job is to Say, "I Love You"

We have been created to love and to be loved.

—MOTHER TERESA

I am a caregiver. My forty-seven-year-old husband, Dave, has a little-known genetic disease called "Huntington's" and can do almost nothing for himself. As a caregiver, I can tell you that we experience a wide range of emotions which largely depend upon the person we are caring for. Lately, I have felt there is really no reward for what I am doing.

Dave has difficulty feeding himself, and swallowing is only accomplished with a great deal of effort. One day, with more food landing on his shirt than in his mouth, David and I were going through the usual "change the shirt" game.

"Dave, lift up your arms," I pleaded. "If you do, we can go and have ice cream."

Dave's garbled speech made his response to my urging impossible to comprehend. I did, however, figure out that he had no intention of lifting his arms or cooperating as I changed the shirt.

I felt myself tense and sighed in frustration. I didn't need this today. Try as I would, I simply couldn't understand what he was saying, and anyway, we weren't moving any nearer our goal—a clean shirt.

"Dave, my job is to feed you, make sure you take your medications, and help your doctors and nurses. Your job is to help me to help you. You need to lift your arms, please."

With an endearing smile so like that of the man I married before the ravages of Huntington's Disease, Dave said, "No. My job is to say, 'I love you,' in as clear a voice as possible."

Caregiving is not something I would ever choose to do. I imagine most people would not choose what is usually an almost thankless job. Especially without pay. But though there may not be pay, there are rewards. Remembering Dave's smile and his "job" is a nice memory I can pull out on days when things get really tough. We all have our jobs, and Dave's job is to say, "I love you."

I love you, too, Dave.

I Love You, Daddy

The cure for all the ills and wrongs, the cares, the sorrows, and the crimes of humanity all lie in the one word, love. It is the divine vitality that everywhere produces and restores life.

—LYDIA MARIA CHILD

═══════════════════

It was unusual that Dave's father, Charlie, was visiting in January. He typically only came to Florida once a year on Dave's birthday in September. Now, here it was, five months since Dave turned forty-eight, and Charlie was not only visiting Florida, but the nursing home as well.

I cannot imagine watching my child go through the myriad of mental, psychological, and physical symptoms that make up Huntington's Disease. No matter how old, how tall, how much grief they cause me, my sons are still my babies and always will be. I know that's how Charlie felt, too.

Dave loves movies, and despite his traitorous body and inability to do anything for himself, he still seems to enjoy our frequent outings to the local theater. What a surprise I got when I walked in to get Dave for our Friday date. Charlie stood talking to Dave's aide by the nurse's station. Charlie, who refused to hear about the home and had a tough time dealing with his son being in such a place, was there with Dave. "Charlie! What are you doing here?"

"Just wanted to congratulate Dave for making it to the year 2000," he replied. "This is a big occasion."

For some reason, and with no warning, he had flown in from Texas to be with Dave and tour the facility. We talked in the car on the way back to Island Lake after seeing the movie *Snow Falling On Cedars*. Well, Charlie and I talked. Dave's speech had gone from difficult to garbled and was now almost non-existent. Despite being able to understand what was going on around him, I had not heard him make more than a few sounds in over six months.

"I need to go back to the car and change my hearing aid batteries," Charlie explained as he walked out of the room once we settled Dave into his wheelchair. "I won't be long."

"Dave, we need to practice while your dad is gone," I pleaded. "Please, Dave. Say, 'I love you, Dad.' I know you can do it."

Dave stared at me intently as he worked his mouth. Meaningless sounds came out, but not the words I knew his father so wanted to hear.

"Dave, I know you can do this. After you say this you never have to talk again if you don't want to, but, please, try as hard as you can. Please?"

With intensity, Dave tried to say the few words that would warm Charlie's heart, but each time he got to the word 'love,' it fell apart. It was just too hard. After several tries, I gave up. Charlie would just have to know in his heart that Dave loved him.

"That's better," said Charlie as he reentered the room. "Now I can hear anything important."

Dave began to shift in his chair and flail his arms.

"Did you want to say something, Dave?" I prompted.

I knew that despite all the changes from Huntington's, Dave was still in there trying desperately to get out. I held my breath and smiled my encouragement.

With effort, Dave slowly but clearly said the four words that I know Charlie heard over and over on his way back to Texas. He broke into a grin as he triumphantly declared, "I love you, Daddy!"

As Charlie knelt to hug Dave in his wheelchair, he buried his face in his son's shoulder. I know the tears he shed were tears of joy from hearing his son proclaim his love.

It's been almost a year since that January day, and Dave has not spoken again. Charlie didn't make the September birthday trek either. He died unexpectedly of an aneurysm three weeks after he hugged his son.

Charlie never gave me a reason for his visit to Florida that January day. He had no way of knowing that he would never again see his son on this earth. I have this picture of Charlie up in heaven, no hearing aid needed, hearing Dave say to him, "I love you, Daddy," and watching his son with all the fatherly pride God intended. And I know God loves them both.

Hope

In all things it is better to hope than to despair.

—JOHANN WOLFGANG VAN GOETHE

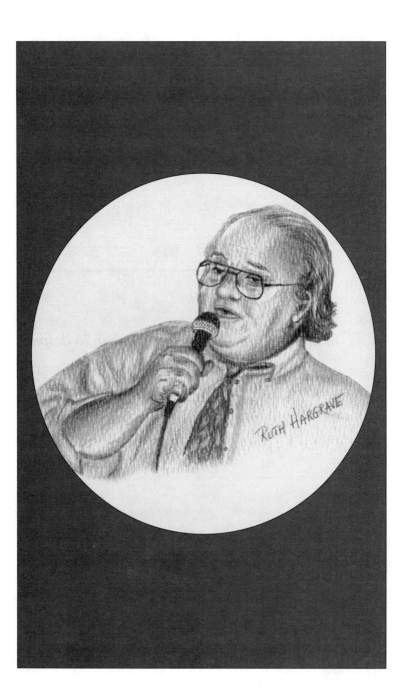

Ruth Hargrave

Passionate Care

What the world really needs is more love and less paperwork.

—PEARL BAILEY

No book that showcases different portraits of Huntington's would be complete without a portrait of one of the many caring professionals who dedicate so much of themselves to the disease. Most of us who each day deal with Huntington's Disease are not here by choice. A flip of the genetic coin is why we are here. Some people, however, *are* here by choice.

Scientists, neurologists, social workers, and others actively choose to be in the thick of the battle, and I, for one, am grateful for their choice. Without them, the level of care would be greatly diminished and the hope for a cure, nowhere on the horizon.

Life is full of lessons, and Jim Pollard learned many of them needed to provide care for families before he had ever heard of Huntington's Disease. Something as seemingly unrelated as being a special education teacher has proven valuable in giving Jim his unique slant on Huntington's Disease and care.

"I worked in special education for twelve years. I taught kids with multiple handicaps, both physical and mental. Most were in their adolescence with a variety of conditions including Cerebral Palsy, Muscular Dystrophy, mental retardation, Autism, specific learning disabilities, and head injuries."

According to Jim, he taught the traditional reading, writing, and arithmetic and a whole lot in between—including toilet training, behavior management, and augmentive communication.

Today, special education programs are the norm in public school systems nationwide, but this was not the case when he started teaching in 1973. "The parents who lobbied for laws to get services for their kids were still very, very active in these classrooms," explains Jim. "I quickly learned that moms knew more about how to deal with and instruct these kids than any textbook or professor."

This important lesson—that families might actually know more than the "experts" when it comes to dealing with those with special needs—is a lesson Jim heard not only in teaching, but also other positions. As the years went by, Jim moved on to manage a special education collaborative for five member towns. His first exposure to the behind-the-scenes management of human services was somewhat discouraging.

"Some, though not a majority of administrators, thought their job description included denying mandated services or, at the very least, making them difficult to get," Jim continues. "Once again I learned from master-moms and crusty old school superintendents how to fight the system or throw a wrench into it. The lessons I learned back then have been invaluable in dealing with the rolls of red tape one needs to cut through with Huntington's Disease."

Jim eventually earned a master's degree. His teaching of special-needs students involved the use of behavior analysis. "Behavior analysis is a liberating technology," says Jim. "For example, one child's mom and I came up with a way to teach severely mentally-handicapped children to use toilet paper. This led to conference and family meeting presentations. It also paved the way for a part-time job teaching teachers in their master's programs."

While Jim loved his job, he also loved his growing family. The responsibilities of raising four children, now ranging from seventeen to twenty-four, required him to look at the financial ramifications of staying in education. Jim knew that without a pHD he was already at the upper end of the salary expectations and would only receive cost of living increases.

About this time, a colleague told him about a job that was open in a nursing home. While Jim had never even thought about working in a nursing home, using his accumulated skills to teach young adults with psychological problems did interest him.

But the residents were middle-aged and had medical conditions that required nursing-home care in addition to various psychiatric conditions. Using basically the same curriculum as he'd used in teaching, Jim took a cut in pay with the likelihood of better pay over time. Thank goodness for us, the gamble paid off because since then, Jim has never stopped working with nursing homes.

Some might call it fate, others coincidence, and still others, God's intervention. Whatever its source, I call it a tremendous break for the Huntington's community.

Six months into the job, Jim got a referral for a patient with Huntington's Disease. He knew little about this disease that strikes both mind and body, only the belief accepted by most nursing homes—that Huntington's Disease candidates were unacceptable for nursing home placement. Jim's acceptance of this popular, albeit erroneous conception, convinced him that their chorea, anger, depression, psychosis, and other symptoms rendered it impossible, and even foolhardy, to even try. But this is where the aforementioned break came in.

The woman who called Jim needed a place where she could get care for her daughter. She refused to believe that *no one* would care for her precious daughter. She refused to accept what others believed. While on the phone, she read Jim the list of symptoms from a National Institute of Health brochure.

"My daughter needs the type of care listed in this brochure," the mother stated. "According to your facility brochure, you offer exactly that type of care. So why won't you take my daughter?"

Hearing this desperate mother speak in such rational, convincing terms, Jim gave in and accepted his first patient with Huntington's Disease. Over the years, there have been hundreds more who have benefitted from Jim's unique slant on accepting and caring for people with both mental and physical symptoms—especially those with Huntington's Disease.

When asked why he continues working with Huntington's Disease families, Jim, never at a loss for words, has this to say: "The rewards I get from helping and coaching a relatively large number of folks in a pitched battle against their HD are greater than I could begin to describe. The level of camaraderie one develops over years of daily challenges is also indescribable. My coaches are family caregivers to whom I listen to intently and from whom I snitch ideas."

"On a more concrete level," Jim continues, "I've been fortunate to have been given these opportunities by the health care executives who support our work as well as a string of colleagues and collaborators." Jim points to Rosemary Best and Sue Imbriglio as two such colleagues. Jim, along with Rosemary, Sue, and a host of others, wrote and compiled *A Caregiver's Handbook for Advanced-Stage Huntington's Disease*. The handbook, a joint initiative of the Huntington's Society of Canada and the Foundation for the Care and Cure of Huntington's Disease, is helping families and care facilities around the world provide the best care possible to those in the latter stages of this disease.

Jim adds that his wife of twenty-five years, Maureen, a delivery room/post-partum nurse, has been beside him every step of the way. His four children, Huntington's families, and co-workers are also all active contributors to his success. "You remove any one of these factors and I couldn't continue, even if I wanted to."

Jim is now the director of the Huntington's Program Laurel Lake Center for Health and Rehabilitation, an eighty-eight bed nursing home in Western Massachusetts. Prior to its opening in May of 1999, Jim was with a home in Lowell, Massachusetts for twelve years. Jim is proud of what has been achieved in under two years and has many hopes and dreams for Laurel Lakes when it comes to HD.

"Today, Laurel Lakes is home to twenty residents with HD. There is also an attached six-bed, assisted-living program for those with HD, with four already filled."

"My goal," Jim continues, "is to provide the best nursing care possible. What that includes is making sure the best nurses, certified nursing assistants (CNA), and others 'get it,' for those with neurologic problems."

According to Jim, perceived "misbehavior" is driven by, or is symptomatic of, the disease. It does not have to do with one's personality, character, or lack of cooperation. "Because the health-care landscape is so stormy these days, my dreams are tempered somewhat by reality. In our case, thankfully, we've been the beneficiary of supportive behind-the-scenes staff in state health care agencies, but that's not always the case. These days, the fate of any health care agency is dependent upon the vagaries of those who pay the bills. The ever-increasing, day-to-day demands put on nursing homes by the regulatory agencies and insurance companies in many cases make simply providing adequate care a stretch. Adequate is not acceptable. Our dream goes way beyond adequate."

Jim Pollard is one of the strongest advocates of care for persons with HD we have. The following is a list he has compiled about providing care until there is a cure. These words show why we need more Jim Pollards on our side.

1. We need to recognize the degree of suffering that is endured by people with Huntington's and their families today. And tomorrow. And the day after that. And probably for days and days after "the cure." Every single day, families touched by HD are screwed by the human service system. They're denied access to existing services they need, they're sent on bureaucratic goose chases, they're locked out of many long-term care facilities, they're victimized by ignorance and enduring myth and misconception. And families are still turning the other cheek! The entire family affected by HD needs to go to their United States senators and congressmen and say, "We're as mad as hell, and we're not gonna take it anymore!"

2. We need to create a democratic national lay advocacy group with leadership elected by the general membership, one that splits the revenue in thirds: direct care, research toward a cure, and political advocacy. The loss of the late Dennis Shea's Foundation for the Care and Cure of HD has drastically reduced the opportunities leaders in care have to discover, collaborate, and disseminate advances in care.

3. Tell your legislators that you're tired of the status quo in nursing homes. You would like them to increase nursing home Medicaid reimbursement. We don't need more nursing home cops. We need more financial resources to attract and keep career caregivers and to reward the ones we already have. We need more people to answer call lights and to help people eat. The relevant maxim is, "You get what you pay for!" We demand better care!

4. Upgrade the curricula of Licensed Practical Nurses (LPN) and the course work required to be a certified nurse aide today. The training in caring for residents with all neurologic conditions, not just HD and dementia, needs improving. Nursing schools, state health departments, regulatory or accrediting agencies... any one of them can initiate this change.

Jim is quick to point out this is not an exhaustive list. "There is more to do, but these are four things that I think of every day—*every single day*."

Looking Beneath the Veil

by Jim Pollard

(Prepared for the Huntington's Disease Association of Ireland
Grand Annual Meeting, Roscommon, May 21, 1999)

*How little do they see what is, who frame their hasty
judgments upon that which seems.*

—ROBERT SOUTHEY

As years go by and Huntington's Disease progresses, it often places a veil over that person you love. He's the same person he always was, it's just difficult to see him through the veil. Sometimes, people who don't really know him or the disease say hurtful things like, "He's a different person," or "He's not the same person he used to be." But understanding some of HD's more subtle aspects will help to lift that veil, and it should come as no surprise that underneath, it is the very same person you have known, loved, and cared for through the years.

Sometimes weakness and changes in facial muscle-tone gives the person with HD a disinterested, even bored appearance—while he may really be laughing on the inside. When greeted by an old friend, for instance, the person with Huntington's will show no expression, appearing less-than-excited about the meeting.

When the old friend asks about his family, because HD makes it difficult to organize thoughts when asked questions, he'll be answered by silence. Just thinking about a simple answer like, "Everyone's fine and my brother's back home now," may take an extra ten seconds. While waiting for the extra ten seconds needed to process the answer in his head, his friend may begin to suspect he's not really interested in conversation or in their reunion.

Other aspects of changes in muscle tone, called "dystonia," may suggest lack of interest in interacting with family and friends. They will often lean over, slouch in chairs, or keep their heads down. Once it is explained that these are aspects of HD, it helps to lift the veil, revealing the person beneath it, as excited as ever to see an old friend!

An impatient family member, one who's insisting on our undivided attention, can be very annoying. In fact, it's very irritating when you count on him to understand how busy you are, but he still insists that you stop what you're doing to attend to him. Can't he see the baby's crying, there's a roast in the oven, and the phone is ringing? Huntington's Disease can certainly make one *appear* selfish, demanding and egocentric. But make no mistake; this is another veil concealing that person that you know as generous or selfless. People with Huntington's often have difficulty controlling impulses and the expression of feelings, especially negative ones directed at you. This creates a very demanding figure. What is worse, damage to certain brain cells means that people with HD just can't wait for anything!

To understand that this impatience is based on a neurologic condition and is not a character flaw helps us to see the person through the veil. While it may not make their unreasonable demands easier to deal with, it does make it more difficult to blame the person under the veil and easier to blame HD.

187

Other aspects of HD tempt us to make negative presumptions about people with Huntington's. Fatigue makes people appear lazy, disinterested, or irritable. Difficulty in controlling movements can make them look drunk, or worse, aggressive. In some instances, their speech has a loud, explosive quality that makes one appear angry. In others, outbursts of anger veils deep depression. All these aspects combine to weave a veil that conceals the person you know so well, and love so much. As we understand and teach others about HD, we are allowed to lift the veil, remove the mask, and see the real person once again. As the Beatles sang, "Look into my eyes now, tell me what you see! It should come as no surprise, what you see is me!"

Cough Drop Cancer

I've seen what a good laugh can do. It can transform tears into hope.

—BOB HOPE

Cancer. The big C. There are few words that evoke such deep-seated dread in the hearer. We all know *someone* who has battled some form of cancer. And even if they beat the monster, it remains a word they never want to hear again.With this in mind, imagine my feelings one middle of the night when I awoke and felt a pain—and a lump—below my arm pit.

"I've got cancer," I thought, fingering the lump under my arm. "It's just not fair. First Dave gets Huntington's Disease, now I get cancer."

The lump felt huge, about the size of a small, oddly shaped marble. I couldn't believe my daily examinations had missed a lump of this size. Of course, I'd spent all my energies meeting Dave or my children's needs, with little time spent on myself. Well, that would have to change.

Like a tongue probing a lost filling in a tooth, I found myself pressing the tender-to-the-touch area. Feeling the sticky lump, I was nearly hysterical. "It's sticky! Oh! It's blood!"

I don't know a lot about cancer, but I do know that bleeding cancer can't possibly be a good thing. My heart raced as I contemplated facing cancer with no insurance. Where would the money come from? Who would take care of Dave? How would my children handle this?

Knowing that I'd never sleep again that night, I decided to read. If I could, that is. First though, I went to the bathroom. I wanted to look into the mirror and see my cancer face-to-lump. But I couldn't. Just couldn't. Seeing it would make it worse somehow. Tomorrow, Scarlet. I'll face this tomorrow.

I returned to my bed as a shaft from the full moon cut across the bed with just enough light to make out a bright red spot on the sheet. Blood. "If it's bleeding enough to make such a dark, intense stain, it must be more advanced than I first realized. This cancer is *advanced*. I've got to confront this," I moaned. I leaned over to touch the red, sticky splotch and then began to laugh, partly in relief, partly in embarrassment.

I've developed allergies since moving to Florida, but I have no insurance. Because of the allergies, I get sinus and ear infections and sore throats. I also read in bed each night before going to sleep, and this night had been no different. I buy cough drops in bulk as I suck on them to soothe my sore throat. It seems I didn't have cancer at all—or my blood had a distinctly cherry smell to it!

Before drifting off, the cherry flavored drop must have fallen onto the bed. Turning over, my flesh pressed against the drop and I slept on it for a number of hours, causing the skin to bruise. The sticky substance stuck to my arm, making it feel as if a lump had formed.

I'm not at risk for Huntington's Disease, nor are my children. I really can't imagine what it must be like to live in a constant state of awareness. For some, every stumble, every forgotten word or temper flare-up signifies the beginning of the end for themselves or their children. It's easy to tell someone, "Don't worry." Human nature, especially if we've seen grandparents, parents, and other family members with symptoms, almost dictates that we worry.

If you or someone you know is at risk, I'm sure you will worry just as I did when I found my "lump." In the midst of your worry, take time to remember that your symptoms might just come from a particularly bad day, parenting teenagers, or the stress of worrying. In other words, your HD might turn out to be as insignificant as my cough drop cancer.

Hope Costs

Hope makes today possible and tomorrow attractive, or at least less threatening. Hope makes death bearable... hope is the mainstay of our energy. We go forward because we hope.

—ARTHUR JONES

The American Heritage dictionary defines hope as, "...a wish or desire accompanied by confident expectation of its fulfillment." I think that's a perfect definition, one we all have to share when we hope for a cure.

Because I am confident my hope will be fulfilled, I tell everyone that I hope for a cure in the near future. I derive this hope from talking to scientists and all I read in medical journals and newspapers.

One day, my son asked me a question. "Mom, if you could have any car you wanted, what would it be?" Now that my sons are of driving age, they talk about cars. *A lot.* Although they know my thoughts on the subject never change, they ask this question time and time again. Without any hesitation, I offer my answer, and it's always the same: "Something that runs, is paid for, and has cheap insurance."

Naturally, they are both appalled, every time. As teenagers, their job is to drool over cars—the faster and shinier, the better. But to me, "those" cars just mean more worries and more expense.

In Hawaii, people had what we called "island" cars. Island cars are covered in rust with paint so badly oxidized it's hard to fathom their original colors. It seemed there were greater numbers of foreign models, but, regardless of the car, they all had one thing in common; you picked them up for a couple hundred dollars and drove them until they died. Eventually, you simply found another one to get from point A to point B.

A few years ago, my older son asked me when he could date. I told him that as soon as he had transportation, he was free to date the prom queen if he so chose. Of course, I then informed him what that meant. "You have to have a license," I advised him. "A license means a 3.5 or better grade point average (GPA) and money for insurance."

"No problem," he smugly assured me. "I have better than a 3.5, and I also have a job."

I dialed my insurance company and handed the phone to him so he could inquire about the cost of a policy for an under-twenty-five-year-old male.

"Yeah, okay. Uh huh… yeah yeah, okay. Thanks."

"So, how much is your insurance, and what's her name?"

"Mom, there is no girl at Lake Mary High School worth that kind of money!"

Nicholas counted the cost and decided it was too high. He didn't date until his senior year. That was when, as an exchange student in the Czech Republic, he quipped, "I have a girlfriend now. We have trains over here."

Nicholas figured it was not worth paying insurance simply to spend more money paying for some girl's portion of the evening. Why, he'd probably never meet her again after graduation. When he arrived in the Czech Republic and counted the revised cost, he decided to date.

There is a cost attached to the hope of finding a cure. Unlike Nicholas, there is no price too dear to pay for eradicating this disease and, as HDSA says, making this the last generation ever to worry about Huntington's Disease. What cost are you willing to pay to fulfill the hope?

There are days when I feel a prisoner to HD. I wake up thinking maybe it's all a bad dream. Anyone else feel that way? Then reality sets in, and I know those thousands of people with HD and those who love them are still being held hostage.

According to Rov Z. Kemp, "There is no better or more blessed bondage than to be a prisoner of hope." On the days I feel like a prisoner, I think about his words. Rather than being held hostage to despair, I choose the bondage of hope.

Sacrifice Fly

Self-sacrifice is the real miracle out of which all the reported miracles grow.

—RALPH WALDO EMERSON

America has a fascination with baseball. I personally find the game about as boring as watching nail polish dry, but then again, I'm not even a nail polish kind of girl.

As long as my father lived, I couldn't bad-mouth baseball in his presence. Lucien Joseph Leal wasn't the first to say or believe it, but he truly felt that baseball was not just a game. Baseball was life.

Some of my childhood memories include watching my dad play softball for the post office or Knights of Columbus leagues. My siblings and I sat in the unrelenting, harsh Kansas sun, bored, wanting to be anywhere but in that treeless park. Who enjoyed watching old men run around bases and strike out? Other old men, we all agreed. But not us.

We'd play with kids under the bleachers, on the swings, or wherever we chose within the perimeters of the invisible fence. We all had to be within viewing distance of the baseball diamond so our parents could see us, and as long as no fights erupted and we behaved, we had some level of freedom.

I don't remember ever seeing a high school or college game, even though the schools I attended allegedly had championship teams. I never saw a professional game until I was almost forty. That's when watching the Baltimore Orioles play the Toronto Blue Jays as a perk of some convention I attended in Baltimore made me question this "baseball is life" metaphor even more. If life is baseball, it must mean life is pretty darned boring.

When David and I dated, he talked about how much he loved sports. In high school, he played football and baseball. Later in life, he enjoyed golf, camping, hiking, and other outdoor activities. *What in the world did he see in me?* I wondered. My sole athletic endeavor came about only because my father demanded I play a few summers on a girls' softball team. I don't remember being the worst player on the team, but memories do fade.

After Dave and I married, he became active in my church until it became his church, too. Men's and couples' Bible studies, serving food at the local mission, and singing in the choir were all activities he enjoyed. They all made him feel a part of the church. But what he *really* liked was the slow-pitch softball team.

For months, all of us wives and girlfriends supported our would-be professionals, watching them vie for the championship against area church teams. We cheered them on to victory as we watched our children and conversed with each other. In the warm Hawaiian sun, with ladies I enjoyed, it wasn't a bad way to spend a Sunday afternoon. However, I still thought baseball was boring, and I still didn't get the "baseball is life" thing. But I was in love, and my new husband's heart beat a little faster each time he looked into the stands and saw me laughing and clapping.

Every team has their star, but none of the contenders for that title feared that Dave might one day rise to the top.

Dave stood firmly at the other end of the spectrum as the worst of these middle-aged jocks.

As each of our men swaggered to the plate, ready to hit one out of the park, we'd each say a silent prayer. "Please don't let him make a fool of himself or, worse yet, get hurt." I'd pray as Dave took his turn. He never seemed upset by his lack of ability, but I was.

He was the catcher, and his teammates were wonderful, cheering every tiny success he had, even the accidental ones. Even when he missed tagging someone out at home, or didn't throw the ball hard enough to reach the pitcher, they didn't give him a hard time.

When Dave and I married, I didn't know he was at risk for Huntington's Disease, though I did find him a bit clumsy. His deteriorating eye-hand coordination, running, and other physical skills, made it increasingly difficult for him to play, but he persevered. With the diagnosis of Huntington's Disease, I understood his lack of ability both on the softball diamond and off.

"You don't have to play on the team anymore if you don't want," I suggested to him after finding out about his illness.

"I want to play," Dave assured me with a grin. "I'm not going to get hurt. Besides, the guys need me. I'm the catcher."

The season wore on with Dave making every game. Every so often he'd get to first base, but more often than not, his awkward, head-first gait slowed him down, with someone tagging him out on second. Still, his optimism stayed intact as we ladies in the bleachers cheered him on.

A curious thing happened during the seasons he played softball. Week after week, as I watched this man I loved so much struggle through each game, I realized, baseball *is* like life. Cleveland Indians' Bob Feller said, "Every day is a new opportunity. You can build on yesterday's success or put its failures behind and start over again. That's the way life is, with a new game every day, and that's the way baseball is."

With Dave, whether playing softball or living life, every new day brought an opportunity to be better than the day before. Softball demanded him to be the best Dave he could be, the best member of his team. Having Huntington's Disease never gave Dave a reason to give up—in baseball or in life.

Baseball is a team sport and so is life. Not one of us on this earth could thrive, or even survive, being alone forever. In the practicalities of life, we'd all fail miserably at growing food, building cars, refining gasoline, or any one of a million other things. Worse yet is the loneliness we'd experience as a "team" of one.

Not one baseball player ever won the game alone. Yogi Berra, Lou Gehrig, Roy Campanella, and even Babe Ruth are all in the hall of fame, in part, because of their teammates. Sure, they had God-given talent and a drive to succeed, but they were just members of a team.

Hank Aaron might have been talking about Dave when he said, "My motto was always to keep swinging. Whether I was in a slump or feeling badly or having trouble off the field, the only thing to do was keep swinging." That's exactly what Dave continues to do even now that he is no longer able to play baseball. He keeps swinging.

During one of Dave's final games, I saw another way that baseball is like life. Bottom of the ninth, scores tied, two outs, bases loaded. We've seen this scenario so often in movies, it's laughable to think that it happened on this day, but it did.

Winning the playoff game meant that the team would advance to the championships. Up at bat? One of the contenders for the "best athlete" award. Swinging the bat as if prepared to hit a home run, the player felt every bit as confident as he looked.

A whispered conversation between the batter and the coach left him shaking his head with a none-to-pleased scowl on his face. It seems the coach instructed him to hit a high pop fly. His posture spoke volumes as he argued with the coach. He could hit a home run, and they'd win by a commanding four points.

The coach patiently explained that they didn't need four points, they only needed one. Every eye remained on the batter as the pitcher wound up, then let loose with that first pitch. Poised on their respective bases, ready to run, three men relaxed as the umpire called, "Ball!"

The batter readied himself. Would the crack of the bat signal a homer or a fly? "Ball two!"

No way would the pitcher walk the guy. If he did, we'd win with just one run, but we'd win. Crack! The bat connected, and they all started their homeward flight. It was a pop fly!

In baseball, there's what is called a "sacrifice fly." A sacrifice fly is a fly ball that enables a runner on third base to score after the ball is caught by a fielder. For the batter, it's an easy out. But, at the bottom of the ninth with the bases loaded, with only one run needed to win, it's the way to go for a team win.

Sure enough, an outfielder, his glove shielding his eyes from the sun, backed farther into the field. He got it! The runner on third, knowing victory depended on his ability to make it home before being tagged out, ran. Yes! We advanced to the championship round!

Watching the drama at play, I finally knew: baseball *is* life. My parents sacrificed much to educate their eight children in private schools and see that they ate nutritious food. They sacrificed their dreams for the team called "family." Teachers sacrificed their own novels or compositions or arts so students could win Pulitzers and Oscars. Military members sacrificed their lives, and team America survived.

Dave no longer plays baseball. He no longer walks or talks or takes care of any of his needs. He is living life and is still part of team Huntington's. To my knowledge, Dave has never asked why *he* was the brother that got Huntington's Disease. He has never quit loving or trusting God, and he has never stopped loving or trusting me. In many ways, Dave is a sacrifice fly.

In a seemingly serendipitous way, Dave and I met and fell in love. I don't think God looked down on us and decided that since Dave would get Huntington's and, because I needed yet more grief in my life, I should meet him. Nor do I think He decided that Dave would need a caregiver and for that reason, orchestrated our marriage. I do believe, however, that nothing is ever wasted in God's economy.

Because I fell in love with a slightly clumsy man who loved baseball, I started to write. Because I write what I know, I write about Huntington's Disease. It is my passion to tell the world and break their hearts so they will give and there will be a cure. I want people to care as much about those with Huntington's as they do about cancer and AIDS and Alzheimer's disease.

I also know there are people in heaven today *because* Dave is a sacrifice fly. Somewhere, there are people who read my writing or hear me when I tell them that God loves them.

When they announce a cure for Huntington's Disease, the scientists will stand and accept accolades and awards, and they will deserve them. I also believe that when we find a cure, and we will, the real heroes are the "sacrifice flies" like Dave. Somewhere out there is a student who read something I've written and now he wants to do research to cure HD. Someone will read this essay and decide to be a sacrifice fly by digging deep and giving their hard-earned money for the cure.

Those in drug studies are sacrifice flies, as are families who donate their departed loved one's brains to science. The list of ways people can sacrifice to find the cure for HD and until then, provide care, is endless. What Frederick B. Wilcox says is true. "Progress always involves risks. You can't steal second base and keep your foot on first."

I can't say I'll ever watch a game of baseball for enjoyment; I still prefer basketball as a spectator sport. I do think about baseball as "life" quite a bit these days, especially when I listen to the news or see a headline about baseball. Of course, when I think about baseball as life, I can't help but think of Dave. My life is richer, and I'm a better person because of my own sacrifice fly.

Endless Dreams

Music is the universal language of mankind.

—HENRY WADSWORTH LONGFELLOW

A few months after the release of *Faces of Huntington's*, I started receiving invitations to speak at Huntington's Disease conferences. Because I was a singer long before I was a writer, it seemed natural to weave meaningful music into my presentations. No matter what is happening in a person's life, no matter how horrible or delightful, I think all people respond to music.

So I began to choose songs with universal appeal. I chose calming, familiar, meaningful songs, and people responded. People asked to take my music home, but I couldn't accommodate their requests. Eventually, I realized that I needed to record a compact disc that accomplished musically what the stories in *Faces of Huntington's* had already managed to communicate.

I sing like I write, cook, and do most things in life; I have no real training, and I don't follow recipes or even many instructions. I do, however, believe in the principle of surrounding myself with excellence. I also believe in prayer. I began to pray that God would provide someone with excellent musical genius to help me create the perfect CD as a companion to the book.

About this time, a lovely woman signed on to the

online Huntington's Disease community, *Hunt-Dis*. Ardith Newbold, better know as Ardie, is a wonderfully articulate woman with three daughters. She also has Huntington's Disease. When I told the group about my plan for recording a project, Ardie quickly responded. "Have you chosen a studio yet?"

"No, I haven't," I answered. "My other projects were all recorded back home in Hawaii. I don't know anyone here in Florida."

"Are you anywhere near Disney? My daughter, Soon Hee, is a musician, and she and her husband, Erin, have a recording studio."

We quickly traded contact information, and I sent Soon Hee an email. A flurry of emails resulted in a meeting. As soon as I met them, I knew they were the ones that I wanted to work with. Besides being incredibly talented, Soon Hee had a passion for creating Huntington's Disease awareness. As she'd been adopted herself, she was not at risk, but having a mother with HD and two at-risk sisters made the disease deeply personal.

Choosing the songs for the CD was the hard part. I wanted songs that captured the essence of each chapter, and I wanted familiar songs that people already loved. There seemed hundreds for each theme! With lots of suggestions from others and hours spent listening to songs, I came up with my final selections. Those talented musicians arranged the music, and the results were better than I ever anticipated.

Erin was a master of patience as we recorded songs over and over in their home studio. With the quality of the recording, it's hard to believe that I actually sang in their closet. Trust me, I did. Even on hot summer days, with the air conditioning off to reduce any noise, I stood amid Soon Hee's dresses and sang.

Then Soon Hee asked if she could write a song for the project. Thrilled, I gave her an enthusiastic "yes." The result was a lovely haunting melody with poignant lyrics. While Huntington's Disease is never mentioned in the song, it turned out to be the perfect song for our cause.

Soon Hee's lyrics challenge us to have endless dreams. Whether it's the dream of a cure, which we all want, or something else, dreams do come true. With Soon Hee's kind permission, I have included the words to "Endless Dreams." Her music is equally special, and some of you have heard me sing it at various HD gatherings. My dream is that each time I sing this song, or each time one of you plays the CD and hears the song, we will come that much closer to having our dream of a cure come true.

I also hope that each of you has your own, personal dreams, and that they all come true.

"Endless Dreams"

Words and Lyrics by Soon Hee Newbold Rettig

Sometimes life is hard to live,
'Cause pain and strife do not forgive.
God gave us hope to make it through the day,
And endless dreams to find a way.

It's sad to think some have no dreams,
Life is lost or so it seems.
Listen to your heart and dare to fly.
We all will fail if we don't try... To have endless dreams.

Chorus

I want to sing from the highest mountain,
Touch the stars in outer space,
Drink from the ageless fountain,
Always see your face.
Why can't we all have endless dreams?

Dreams create our destiny,
And we know with certainty.
Through all the laughter and all the tears,
We'll find a cure for our worst fears.
And have endless dreams.

Chorus

Bridge

Your life is part of a greater plan,
Only He knows why this began.
Just remember when it's too much to cope,
There is endless hope

Chorus (twice)

For more information about the *Faces of Huntington's* CD, please visit http://www.writerspeaker.com or call 1-800-431-1579.

Joy

---

*Real joy comes not from ease or riches
or from the praise of others, but from
doing something worthwhile.*

—WILFRED GRENFEL

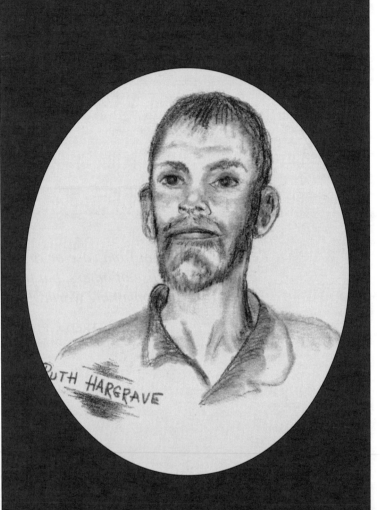

The Essence of a Life

We are here to add what we can to life, not to get what we can from it.

—WILLIAM OSLER

"How long has Dave been sick?" people ask. That's a hard question to answer. I wish I could tell you every detail about Dave's life, but I can't. Both of his parents have passed away, and his brother has not been in communication with me. He does have cousins and other family members, but, like so many families, it seems it's easier for them to live their lives and ignore someone who is sick. I guess I understand. It just makes me sad.

I do know that Dave was born in Oklahoma on September 4, 1951, and that his parents divorced when he was around nine years old. His mother eventually remarried and moved to Pennsylvania with her new husband. As I understand it, Dave's younger brother, Daryl, spent more time with his mother, while Dave stayed with his father.

Before we ever knew that Huntington's Disease was in our future, I once asked Dave how he could be such an even-tempered man. Nothing seemed to faze him, and there was always a solution to every problem. I loved that about him.

He told me his father lost his temper a lot and yelled. Dave vowed that he would never be like his father, and for the most part, he kept that vow. Of course, I noticed that

Dave had more of his father in him than he liked to admit.

Dave's father, Charlie, had a significantly higher-than-average IQ. Charlie served as the president of the Oklahoma chapter of Mensa, an organization for people whose IQ is in the top 2 percent of the population. Dave may not have wanted to have his father's temperament, but he inherited much of his father's intelligence.

Dave struggled with learning, mostly due to his dyslexia, but he still managed to obtain his Master's of Business Administration. He had a broad interest in a variety of subjects. My children loved to test his knowledge and were constantly amazed at how much he knew about so many varied topics.

Dave also inherited his father's stubbornness and tenacity. When Dave was young, he had a paper route. When they discover how difficult the job is, most kids give up quickly, or at least once school activities start to take over. Not Dave. He had that route all the way through high school because he had a goal. First, he wanted, and bought, a bicycle with his earnings. After that, he worked to earn enough for a school trip to Washington, D.C.

His tenacity didn't let him quit football or trumpet lessons either. Once Dave started something, he never gave up.

Dave and his first wife married right after high school, then relocated to Phoenix, Arizona, where her mother lived. When people learn that he has two children, Andrew and Jessica, they ask if they have the gene, too. I hope they don't, but as letters, cards, and phone calls all went unanswered after his first wife was informed of Dave's diagnosis, with all its ramifications, I can't say. I do know that when I talk about them to Dave, his eyes still sparkle and he smiles. He remembers and loves his children.

I first met Dave when, after his divorce, he moved to Hawaii to stay with his father and stepmother. We met at a Parents Without Partners meeting. I didn't want to go, but a friend begged and pleaded, so I gave in. She ended up a no-show, but I met Dave. The rest, as they say, is history.

Dave might have inherited intelligence, stubbornness, and tenacity from his father, but he inherited the gene for Huntington's Disease from his mother. Unfortunately, a misdiagnosis of Multiple Sclerosis is the reason Dave never knew he was at risk for HD.

Looking back, now that I have learned so much about this disease, I think Dave probably had symptoms before I ever met him. The age of HD onset is puzzling to many, including those in the medical profession. In some cases, particularly when there is significant chorea, the emergence of physical problems makes it easier to pinpoint when symptoms began.

Dave has little chorea, or uncontrollable movements, and is more rigid. His first symptoms were mental rather than physical. I've heard it said that Huntington's takes a person's personality traits and exaggerates them. This may not be true in all cases, but it describes Dave perfectly.

What I first saw as stubbornness inherited from his father, magnified until, within eighteen months of our marriage, my sweet husband had changed. His previous quirk of setting tomorrow's clothing out each night became a compulsion. The 6:30 dinner was etched in stone, and life as we knew it would end if it changed.

Walking on eggshells may be a cliché, but it really applies to the life that we all lived before we knew of Dave's illness. My sons could no longer laugh loudly because it upset him. He dictated not only our meal times, but our television viewing habits, our activities, and more. A frightening paranoia kicked in, making life "interesting," to say the least.

Dave's behavior *could* have been because he was trying to parent two stepsons. It *could* have been the new job or settling into a new marriage. Looking back, I chalked his behavior up to a mid-life crisis, culture shock from living in Hawaii, and many other things. Then came the physical symptoms.

Rapid weight loss, frequent falling, swallowing problems, and other obvious symptoms eventually triggered a series of events that culminated in a diagnosis of Huntington's Disease. In many ways, I think Dave was relieved. His tenacious spirit had pushed him along, despite what his body and mind were doing. Now he could relax.

In the final chapter of *Faces of Huntington's*, I included a list written by Jim Pollard and Rosemary Best. *The Alternative Stages of Huntington's Disease* allows us to look at the various stages in positive terms from the point of view of the person with Huntington's Disease.

Rereading this priceless piece, I thought about how it applied to Dave, who is in the final stage of Huntington's. I'm sure you could each personalize the stages by thinking about someone you know with HD.

The Alternative Stages of Huntington's Disease According to David Pock

Defiance: "I'm not denying the diagnosis, I'm defying the verdict! I'm not refusing to accept it, I'm just boldly resisting the inevitable!"

Once we understood about Huntington's Disease and its effect on Dave and the family, I wondered, would Dave give up? I read that some people do deny the diagnosis, but not Dave. Not only did he refuse to deny the diagnosis, he went with me to our first HDSA convention in Philadelphia. Seeing others with Huntington's actually empowered him.

We jointly decided to start a support group back home in Hawaii, and when I decided to write my first book, we talked openly about telling others about him and our lives. Dave always felt helping others learn about this disease, and how to cope with it, made living with Huntington's more tolerable.

When I speak locally for United Way or other organizations, Dave comes with me. Even though he can no longer speak, he is communicating volumes simply by his willingness to attend.

Perseverance: "I'm continuing on... in spite of all the difficulties this damn disease puts in front of me."

In true form, Dave accepted his reality and went about his life unwilling to cave in. He still went to Bible study and played on the church softball team. He continued interacting with friends and best of all, his faith continued to grow.

Of course, as the symptoms worsened, it became obvious that we needed to seek the right medication. Sadly, Dave's resolve not to be like his father was not to be. Unreasonable requests and expectations soon turned into yelling, and even physical violence. I knew it was the disease that made Dave violent, but it still hurt to see him like that. Finally, the second time he tried to kill my son, I understood that we had reached a new level.

Compassion: "I'm sorry for the trouble I'm causing my family and everyone else who cares for me. I wish I could do something to help them."

213

To some degree, the medication brought my Dave back to me. Yes, there were still outbursts but, more often than not, peace returned to our house. During this time, he accepted the feeding tube his doctor suggested and also the swallowing specialist. I can remember Dave apologizing for how expensive everything was. His food and medication gobbled up our monthly income and he felt badly. I quickly assured him that everything works out somehow, and each month it did.

Moving 5,000 miles from home created difficulties for all of us. Even though he never voiced his thoughts, I know it must have been hard for him to move from where he had friends or family. But he never complained and enjoyed life as best he could.

Stamina: "I'm not sure just what it is but something keeps me going! It keeps me going through all my fatigue and all the problems and hardship this damn disease presents me."

Dave always said that he only wanted the feeding tube until his quality of life changed to the point at which he didn't want to continue anymore. Only Dave could choose that point. When he decided the time was right, he yanked out his tube and took it to the nurse. Without calling me, or following the instructions written on his chart, the nurse reinserted Dave's tube.

Unable to voice his thoughts, Dave let his anger speak for him; he began hitting other residents and staff in the nursing home where he now lives. It took me a while to figure out the source of his anger, because he still received the same medication as before his recent behavior change. Eventually, though, I realized the problem. After several discussions, the tube was permanently removed.

A few months later, Dave returned to eating by mouth again. The nursing-home administrator said to me, "You were right and we were wrong. We all gave Dave a couple of months at most. You knew exactly what he wanted."

Somehow, through the problems and fatigue, Dave keeps going on. Something in him won't give up.

Grace: "I've quietly resigned myself to needing others to care for me, to sustain me. I can't show them, but I'm more concerned for the welfare of those around me than I am for myself. We know we're there for each other."

The other day I went to visit Dave, as I do several times each week. On this day, he was in the day room by the nursing station. Two of the aides were doing reports and talking to him. He couldn't answer, but his presence added much to the room.

"Dave's our favorite," they each proclaimed.

They say he's great company, especially when he smiles. That morning, I mentioned Dave's new haircut and reminded him that Wendy cut his hair. An ear-to-ear grin brightened his face.

"Dave has an eye for the women," I explained. Wendy is cute and bubbly and hugs Dave and treats him special. Just hearing her name makes him happy.

Dave never complains about anything these days. His grace and acceptance in a terrible situation shines through.

When I met Dave, I was struck by how comfortable he was with himself as a person and as a man. He genuinely liked himself and his happiness didn't depend on material wealth or what others thought of him.

How do you sum up the essence of his forty-nine

years? I can do it in one word… joy. Dave found and kept his joy though acquiring knowledge of the disease, always enjoying and bringing laughter into his and others' lives, and demonstrating patience. He continues to show compassion for those around him, has never lost his strong faith, is generous with his love and knows he is loved. He never gives up hope.

If I could have one wish, it wouldn't be for a cure for Huntington's Disease. We wouldn't need a cure, because I would wish that Huntington's Disease never existed.

I can't make that wish come true, so I'll have to be content with knowing I've learned many valuable lessons since hearing about Huntington's Disease. Dave has helped me to actively choose joy in my life. I am a better person for being a joyful person, and so is Dave.

She's Prettier

Recollection is the only paradise from which we cannot be turned out.

—JEAN PAUL RICHTER

Dave loves movies. Action, drama, comedy, it doesn't matter—as long as it's not horror. Now that there are so many things he cannot do, I make sure to take him to see a movie three or four days a week. It's the least I can do, and as long as I can transfer him, I'll keep doing it.

One day, we'd settled down to enjoy *Blast From the Past*, starring Brendan Fraser and Alicia Silverstone. I've gotten to the point where I don't expect much from a movie. They seem to be either all made from the same template or riddled with profanity, gratuitous sex, and violence. But surprisingly, this was a movie I liked.

"I need to go to the bathroom," Dave said. It took an effort to figure out what Dave wanted; his verbal skills are increasingly worsening. He tried to rise, and I realized that yes, he did need to go to the bathroom. Since he can still walk and function reasonably well, I wanted to give him the dignity of going unaided.

After a few scenes though, I realized that Dave had been away longer than going to the bathroom warrants. As hard as it was, I tore myself away from the man born in a bomb shelter who had suddenly been exposed to modern-day society, and went out to find Dave.

I poked my head into the mens' room and yelled his name, to no avail. Nothing but silence was in that room. I tried the ladies' room, too, with the same effect. The Wednesday matinee doesn't bring many people to our suburban theater.

After searching the lobby, I approached the teenager behind the concession stand. "Have you seen Dave? You know, the tall guy I come to the movies with," I asked.

With the practiced shrug only a teenager can accomplish, he said, "No."

"Would you please call the manager?"

He stared at me, then shrugged again and picked up and mumbled into the walkie-talkie. I scanned the lobby again, hoping against hope that Dave would appear before the manager arrived. No luck.

When the theater manager appeared, she explained that she'd looked for Dave in the ticket booth, and the projection room. I didn't wait to explain that he couldn't possibly have climbed the stairs. I thanked her, then rechecked both restrooms again, the store room, and every possible place in the theater. No Dave.

Lake Mary Cinema has eight theaters; I decided to check into each one. Maybe, I reasoned with myself, he'd simply gone into the wrong one.

With renewed optimism, I began on my left and entered the first theater. When going to the movies, Dave and I always sit in exactly the same place so he won't get lost coming back from the bathroom. One by one, I walked into each theater, looked at the back row, left-hand side, and continued down the first aisle and up the next, trying unobtrusively to spot Dave.

Until then, I'd managed to keep a cool head. But as I exited the last theater, heading toward the lobby again, I began to panic. I realized that he had most likely gone outside. I knew I had to get help, which meant I needed the police.

Under two minutes later, two police officers entered the lobby. I explained that Dave was outside, alone, and, giving them the shortest crash course on Huntington's Disease I could manage, explained why it was so unsafe for him to be outside alone. I told them that, besides his unsteady gait, he can't communicate well and has poor judgement. "We need to find him as soon as possible," I said, trying to keep the tremble out of my voice.

"Why don't you go back and watch your movie. If your husband comes back there and you're gone, he'll probably panic. We'll walk through this strip mall and see if he's in any of the shops."

I gave them a physical description and whipped out a photo of Dave, explaining that he had lost a huge amount of weight since the picture. This led to part two of my HD 101 lesson to help them really understand the odds.

"What happens if he isn't in any of the shops?" I asked.

"We'll most likely find him. But if not, we'll show his picture on the TV during the six and ten o'clock news and ask for help. Probably put up the helicopter, too."

Oh great! That's all I needed. The picture I had given the police, taken three years previously, included my sons. If they used the picture, sixteen-year-old Justin would go ballistic. Nick was safely away in college, but Justin would be beyond embarrassed. He'd be livid. Having a stepfather with a terminal disease was bad enough. Having the entire five-county area learn about it would be a disaster in Justin's mind.

Since my first book came out, Justin's biggest fear is that somehow I'll be on Oprah. Not being one to pass up a chance to even a score, I told him to be afraid, very afraid. "*When,* not *if,* I'm on Oprah, I'll wear a tight-fitting black T-shirt." I went on, eye-to-eye with my disbelieving off-spring, "the huge white letters covering my chest will pro-claim, "I'm Justin's mom."

Okay, so the Central Florida news is not Oprah, but his friends might see the news. Horrors! Now I had two wor-ries: Dave's safety and the wrath of Justin, should the SWAT team take to the air.

Back in my seat, I found it impossible to concentrate on the movie. I couldn't stop my mind from racing, worry-ing.Where was Dave? Was he okay?

Finally, after 45 more nerve-wracking minutes, the credits rolled and the film ended. I readied myself for the news that Dave had not been found and tried to think what to do next. Picking up my purse and Dave's jacket, I turned towards the door only to see Dave walking toward me. He was safe! But where were the policemen?

As I entered the lobby, the manager and two policemen approached us. "He's fine, Ma'am," the younger officer assured me.

It seems that Dave had never been outside at all. He'd been in the theater right next to ours. He was watching *Simply Irresistible* with Sarah Michelle Gellar.

"Why didn't you come back?" I asked. Dave looked for all the world like a young kid caught with his hand in a cookie jar. "We saw that movie yesterday."

"She was prettier."

Dave might have Huntington's Disease but he's still a guy. He thinks Sarah Michelle Gellar is prettier than Alicia

Silverstone. That's that. Besides, Dave wasn't lost at all. As I searched the bathrooms and talked to the staff, Dave must have been trying to find the right movie. Evidently, he sat down after I had already passed his seat, and that's why I couldn't find him when I searched the theaters. He wasn't worried at all. He was too busy enjoying Sarah Michelle.

I guess, from now on, we have to choose our movies based on leading ladies. The most important thing is that Dave enjoys our outings. They say that people with Huntington's don't lose their memories, they just have a hard time communicating those thoughts. I sincerely pray that when Dave can no longer go out and see movies, and he can no longer talk about things, he will remember the women from all the movies we've seen. He deserves nice memories.

Dave's Goofy Day

The best portion of a good man's life is his little, nameless,
unremembered acts of kindness and of love.

—WILLIAM WORDSWORTH

Tuesday, February 24, 1998 is more glorious than I could have anticipated. In the aftermath of the terrible Central Florida storms, the picture-perfect day is a gift. Not only is it welcome respite for those who have lost their homes in the devastating level-four tornadoes, it is an answer to prayer for Dave.

My husband, Dave, loves Goofy. No, let me replace "loves," with the word, "obsesses." What Dave feels for Goofy is definitely bordering on obsession. For Christmas I gave him his heart's desire: two Goofy shirts that he wears almost exclusively. It's no surprise that the last thing on Dave's "to do" list is to visit Disney World.

At forty-six years of age, Dave shuffles through his days like an old man of eighty. As his appetite and ability to swallow continue to decrease, so does his weight. Sometimes I am not sure who lives in his body: the three-year-old child or the old man who sits and stares into space. On this day, there is no question; it is the three-year-old, dressed in his purple Goofy shirt, eager to go to Disney World.

I could never afford Disney tickets for my family of four, but I want to give Dave a special day. In the last stage of Huntington's, I know time is running out. Thanks to the generosity of the wonderful Disney Compassion Program, we are going to make a memory.

As excited as Dave is about the excursion, I have a nagging concern. What if we get to the park and Goofy can't be found? But no need to worry! Look! There's Goofy, right inside the front gate, holding court with dozens of young fans clutching their autograph books, faces glowing as they excitedly wait to greet their favorite character. I wheel Dave's chair up the ramp and wait behind the children, none of them older than five. I alternate between feeling happy for Dave, embarrassed because of his obvious age and disability, and unbearably sad for myself at the loss of my dreams. Before Huntington's Disease ravaged his brain, Dave earned a Master's of Business Administration degree. Dave is himself a parent, yet now, the crowning achievement in his life is to spend time with Goofy.

It's Dave's turn. His face is one incredibly ecstatic smile and Goofy seems to know he's special. Instead of the brief time spent with the kids, Dave gets a hug, a caress on the arm with the floppy ear, a kiss on the cheek, posing for pictures, and another hug. A lady with a Polaroid camera takes a picture for Dave to carry around all day, since our photos will need developing. I am trying hard to smile, but it's difficult to breathe as I watch Dave's childlike delight through a blur of tears.

A turquoise Goofy shirt and colorful Goofy doll are a necessity, and every few minutes, Goofy comes out of the bag and Dave talks to him and beams. Dave's wheelchair gets the royal treatment, and there are no lines for us as we breeze through the park. Dave and Goofy enjoy every ride, even the scary ones. It is truly a perfect day.

Tonight, Dave sleeps with Goofy and wakes me to find the doll whenever it gets tangled in the covers, or falls to the floor. I know when the hospice workers come tomorrow, he will trip over his words as he excitedly relates the story of his day and Goofy to them.

He told me this morning that now, since he got to meet Goofy, God can call him home so he can see the angels in heaven. I think Dave has already seen some angels. I am convinced that Donna with Disney Compassion Program and the employee in the Goofy suit are angels. Only an angel would treat Dave with such dignity and joy on his extraordinary day. The caring lady, conveniently standing nearby with a Polaroid, just has to reside in heaven.

Part of me is happy to give Dave his Goofy day, and the other half is in mourning for the husband I thought I had already said goodbye to years ago. I feel a loss as I have not felt since he was first diagnosed. Sometimes I wonder how I can ever survive, but I know God will continue to bring angels alongside me whenever I really need them. He always does.

The Hair Train

Memory is the diary we all carry about with us.

—OSCAR WILDE

My father believed that girls should have long hair. I think if my mother had been able to cast the deciding vote, her four daughters would have had pixie or pageboy cuts. She struggled each morning to tame four wild heads into appropriate hairstyles.

Tender headed. That's what Mamma called me. With a head full of naturally curly hair, I'm sure I endured more pain than my three sisters combined. They had obedient, straight hair, easily subdued into two long plaits suitable for Catholic school. I, on the other hand, had defiant hair. So, each morning the cries could be heard from the house on Munson Avenue, until finally, my hair passed muster and off we went.

As much as my mother must have dreaded the morning hair-combing ritual, she hated washing all that hair even more. I once asked my mother if she preferred parenting boys or girls. Without hesitation she said, "If I could do it again and I had a choice, I'd have eight boys instead of four of each." Thanks, Mamma. Of course maybe it's because my brothers had hassle-free, easy-to-wash hair.

My mother expressed creativity in how she got our hair washed. I can still see four little girls, trudging in the hot, humid Kansas heat, downtown to the beauty school.

With the huge dryers and the crush of ladies, the air inside the beauty school was not much cooler than the temperature outside. At least we could sit down and wait for the unfortunate students assigned to unsnarl and wash our tangled locks.

Diane particularly hated our sometimes weekly excursions to the beauty school. She always seemed to get stuck with the student who knew the least about braiding hair. Invariably her braids would be lopsided, and we'd have to wait until they were, if not perfect, at least presentable.

My mother had a certain set of rules we were supposed to live by, and she would ask the same question when we collapsed after our four-mile round trip. Mamma would ask, "Were you drinking Coke when you were walking home?"

We could honestly tell her no. We really weren't drinking Coke from the beauty school. We'd collect abandoned pop bottles on the way there and, on the way home, stop and turn them in for enough money to buy two bottles of pop that we'd proceed to share. We made sure to get orange or grape or even some sort of lemon-lime. Never Coke. We laughed about that little unladylike deception for years.

Our favorite way to get our hair washed, though, was Aunt Cia. Her name was Cecilia, and she wasn't our real aunt, but to us, she was family. Aunt Cia lived around the corner and down the alley. On nice summer days, Mamma sent us over to Aunt Cia to have our hair washed.

She'd patiently work through the jungle of tangles and knots and wash our hair before sending us out to the yard. The four of us sat on a large blanket, usually in chronological order. Debbie, two years my elder, sat cross-legged while

I brushed her cocoa locks with long, rhythmic strokes. Diane, two years my junior, tugged her wide-toothed comb through my spiral curls, while Patricia, predictably two years younger still, worked on Diane's thick, brown mane.

After ten minutes of girl-talk, punctuated by shrill giggles, Patricia would cry, "When's it my turn?" The all-girl locomotive would change direction with Debbie taking on the caboose role as Diane brushed Patricia's silky tresses.

Aunt Cia's laundry billowed in the soft breeze, drying under the scorching sun in the cloudless Kansas sky. Back then, with no thoughts of skin cancer or wrinkles, we enjoyed our respite from chores and brothers as we chuckled and snickered and sometimes even shrieked with laughter.

With our freshly-washed hair smelling like the shampoo on television where a pearl made its way to the bottom of the bottle, we trooped into Aunt Cia's kitchen. Lunch always consisted of condensed tomato soup served in blue or pink plastic bowls, with a pat of butter on top. I hated that butter, and never waited for it to melt, but threw it on the grass as we made our way back to the patchwork blanket.

I never thought about what a sacrifice Aunt Cia made all those Saturdays. She had a mentally-challenged son, but she still made room in her schedule to wash our hair and make our lunch. What an incredible break for my mother! And what a bonding time for us sisters.

I hope each of you has an Aunt Cia in your life. Someone who watches your loved one while you run out. Or maybe brings over dinner on one of those tough days when cooking is the last thing you can think about. It could be a person who just lets you talk until you're all talked out.

227

I don't know if my mother ever thanked Aunt Cia for the countless Saturdays. I know I certainly didn't. She's gone now, but I hope she knows how much I appreciated her. I also hope that you make it a point to thank the Aunt Cias in your life.

The Joyful Generation

Know that joy is rarer, more difficult, and more beautiful
than sadness. Once you make this all important discovery,
you must embrace joy as a moral obligation.

—ANDRE GIDE

The American Heritage dictionary defines the word generation as "a group of individuals born and living about the same time." It is only recently that generations have been given catchy names such as the "Baby Boomers," "Baby Busters," and "Generation X."

In his 1998 book, NBC news anchor Tom Brokaw chronicles what he calls "The Greatest Generation." In this collection of stories from veterans and others from the WWII era, Brokaw "salutes those whose sacrifices changed the course of American history." As inspiring as these stories are, there's another generation Brokaw's book does not cover; a generation with the opportunity to impact lives throughout the world.

The Last Generation. That's the rallying cry from the Huntington's Disease Society of America. In the award-winning HDSA video, "Generation 2000," various members of the HD family point out the desire for this to be the last generation that will ever have to worry about Huntington's Disease. Thanks to researchers, there is now tremendous hope that this really *will* be the last generation.

My question is, how will *you* help make sure this is the last generation? It's easy to place the responsibility on others. Maybe you think of yourself as an "only." Your excuse might be that you're too young, too old, too busy, only at risk, only a caregiver. None of the above will get you off the hook, because we need *everyone* to make a difference.

With Dave's diagnosis of Huntington's Disease, I went through the full range of emotions. Like you, when you got a diagnosis about yourself or someone you love, I was sad, depressed, perplexed, and finally, angry. Why David? He was a good person who never hurt anyone. Why my family? None of us deserved this. The truth is, no one deserves to have Huntington's Disease in their family, but that is small consolation for those who daily have to deal with the reality of this long-term neurological nightmare. And it's small consolation to their family and friends as well.

Once we knew that the diagnosis was not a mistake, I decided to read as much as possible about Huntington's Disease. I wanted to know everything about how others deal with the myriad issues surrounding HD. I grew still angrier when I realized how very little was written about the people whose lives were affected, whether they actually had HD, were at risk, or were caregivers.

Three years later, there have been a few more books published, an explosion of information available through the Internet, more people who are willing to talk about Huntington's, more money has been raised, and we are closer to a cure. And there is still no cure.

Clare Boothe Luce once said, "There are no hopeless situations; there are only people who have grown hopeless about them." Are you one of those people?

Every breathing human being is born into an ongoing journey traveled throughout a lifetime. There are many courses that steer our journeys in many directions.

Whether you have Huntington's Disease or are involved for another reason, life is a journey. The question is, is your journey a journey of joy? Turning your life's journey into a journey of joy is a process.

We all make choices daily. As I wrote in the preface, "When we actively pursue knowledge, laughter, patience, compassion, faith, love, and hope, we are in a better position to choose joy." Whatever our choice, it will change the course of our journey, making a difference in how our lives touch others. If we choose joy, we are placed in a position to make that difference a positive one. Joyful people are never hopeless people.

Never consider yourself an "only." The more you choose joy, the more you will understand how important your unique contribution is to achieving our goals. Joy is a choice that helps you to continue having hope.

I believe with all my heart that we are the last generation to suffer with Huntington's. I also believe that our hopes have a better chance of being realized if we are the joyful generation.

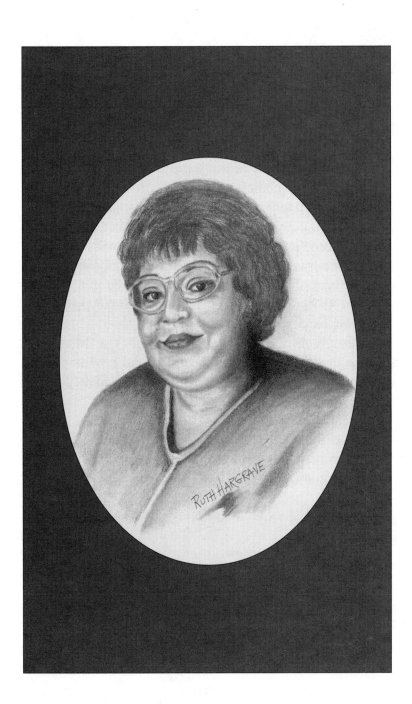

About the Author

Carmen Leal is the author of *Faces of Huntington's* (Essence, 1998), a book for, and about, people with Huntington's Disease and others who care. She is the co-author of *Pinches of Salt, Prisms of Light* (Essence, 1999), a collection of writings about ordinary people doing extraordinary things. Her writings have been featured by *Focus on the Family*, *Decision Magazine*, *William Morrow*, *Simon and Schuster*, *Broadman and Holman*, the *Orlando Sentinel*, and numerous national and local publications.

Carmen is also the author of *WriterSpeaker.com* (Shaw Books, 2000) an Internet research and marketing guide for writers and speakers. She is currently working on a novel and screenplay called *Magic Bullet*.

In addition to her writing, Carmen is a professional speaker and singer. A storyteller with a dramatic testimony, she is a popular presenter at conventions, conferences, and church groups throughout the United States. Carmen is known for her down-to-earth style and common-sense approach to dealing with life, as well as her enthusiasm and sense of humor.

In addition to her Huntington's and inspirational programs, she teaches workshops on topics such as, "The Internet for Writers and Speakers," "Marketing for Writers and Speakers," "Self-Publishing," and "Writing for Publication" at national writers' conferences, churches, bookstores, and writers groups.

About the Artist

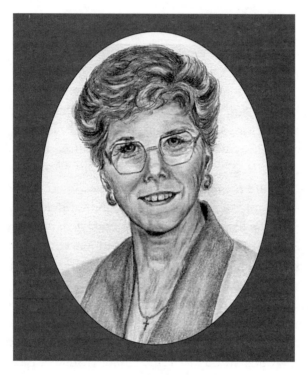

Ruth Hargrave is a member of the National Decorative Painters Association, the Tidewater Decorative Painters, and sits on the Currituck Senior Center Board. She has earned five gold medals and one silver in seven county art competitions.

Ruth is active in Huntington Disease fund-raising, attends the local support group meetings, and was a featured speaker at the 2000 national HDSA convention in Orlando and the HD Symposium in Newport News, VA.

Appendix

Resources on Huntington's Disease

There are an increasing number of resources for families dealing with Huntington's Disease. A large variety can be found through various HD associations throughout the world. Listed below are three starting-points, If you need information for other countries, any of these organizations can guide you to international groups.

The Hereditary Disease Foundation

11400 West Olympic Boulevard Suite 855
Los Angeles, CA 90064-1560
(310) 575-9656 Fax: (310) 575-9156
http://www.hdfoundation.org
E-mail: cures@hdfoundation.org

Huntington's Disease Society of America (HDSA)

158 West 29th Street 7th Floor
New York, NY 10001-5300
(1-800) 345-HDSA Fax: (212) 239-3430
http://www.hdsa.org
E-mail: hdsainfo@hdsa.org

Huntington's Society of Canada (HSC)

151 Frederick Street Suite 400
Kitchener, Ontario N2H 2M2

(519) 749-7063 Fax: (519) 749-8965
Toll Free in Canada: 1-800-998-7398
http://www.hsc-ca.org
E-mail: info@hsc-ca.org

The Internet provides a wealth of information for those who have access to online services. The premiere site online today, for information regarding resources both online and off, is the Hereditary Disease Advocacy Center. Their tremendous site features links to the vast majority of sites on the Internet.

Huntington's Disease Advocacy Center

http://www.hdac.org

Brain and Blood Donations

The donation of a brain or blood from a person with HD is a tremendous gift of hope to research and future generations. For more information on brain tissue donation, write or call:

Harvard Brain Tissue Resource Center

Hereditary Neurological Disease Center
Greg Suter, Director
654 N Woodchuck St.
Wichita, KS 67212
(316) 721-9250

McLean Hospital, 115 Mill Street
Belmont, MA 02178-9106
(800) 272-4622

National Neurological Research Bank

Dr. Wallace W. Tourelotte, Director
West Los Angeles VA Medical Center
11301 Wilshire Blvd.
Los Angeles, CA 90073
(310) 268-3536

To bank blood samples call or write:

Bank by Mail Program
National HD Roster Project
Indiana University Medical Center
975 West Walnut Street
Indianapolis, IN 46202-5251
(Call collect) General: (317) 274-2241
DNA Bank: (317) 274-5745
HD Roster: (317) 274-5744

Order Form

If you have found this book helpful, you might consider ordering a copy for a family member, friend, neighbor, pastor, or a member of the medical profession. Only by telling our story can we raise awareness and funds to help find a cure.

Name: _____

Address: _____

City: _____ State/Prov.: _____

Zip/Postal Code: _____ Telephone: _____

_____copies @ $16 US / $21 Cdn.: $_____

Shipping: ($3.00 first book – $1.00 each add. book) $_____

Florida residents add 7% Sales Tax: $_____

Total amount enclosed: **$**_____

Payable by Check or Money Order

International orders can be processed through Amazon.com with a credit card. If you prefer paying by check, please send in US funds. US and Canadian orders may also call 1-800-431-1579.

Send to: *Portraits of Huntington's*
Living Hope, Inc.
P.O.Box 9426
Naples, FL 34101-9426

Volume discounts are available as a fundraiser to associations and chapters. Please inquire for special pricing information. For more information about the *Portraits of Huntington's,* please email: Carmen@writerspeaker.com, or http://www.writerspeaker.com.